Resilience and Posttraumatic Growth of Breast Cancer Survivors

Abstract

Although there is an abundance of information in the literature pertaining to breast cancer resiliency and posttraumatic growth, research on the impact of early-life experiences that either promote or detract from psychological growth in survivorship is lacking. This study investigated whether resiliency and posttraumatic growth determined from some types of abusive experiences during childhood mediate further growth when confronted with subsequent traumatic experiences in adulthood, specifically breast cancer treatment/survival. Data were collected through participant self-report of information using a retrospective questionnaire on perceived childhood discipline and abuse, resiliency, and posttraumatic growth. Specifically, the Emotional and Physical Abuse Questionnaire (EPAB) served as the abuse measure. The Predictive 6-Factor Resilience Scale (PR6) was used to measure resilience, while the Posttraumatic Growth Inventory (PTGI) measured posttraumatic growth. Results revealed that mild and severe physical abuse as well as greater degrees of emotional abuse were significantly positively associated with posttraumatic growth. Emotional abuse was associated with resilience specifically when survivors experience a sense of physical and emotional wellbeing, while physical abuse was not associated with resilience even when considering wellbeing factors.

Keywords: breast cancer, resiliency, posttraumatic growth, childhood abuse, trauma

Table of Contents

List of Appendices

List of Tables

List of Figures

CHAPTER ONE: INTRODUCTION

The chances of developing breast cancer in a woman's lifetime are 1 in 8, and breast cancer is the second leading cause of cancer death in women (Niakan et al., 2021). Learning of a breast cancer diagnosis comes as a shock to most women, as they are immediately confronted with the fear of loss of life, changes in body image, and apprehension regarding the aggressive nature of treatment (Loeffler et al., 2018). As cancer care begins, worry tends to intensify, and rigorous treatment may also result in symptoms of depression. Following treatment conclusion, some survivors continue to experience anxiety and distress as related to a variety of issues including fear of mortality and altered body image (Andrykowski et al., 2008).

In the long term, however, many breast cancer survivors learn to adapt, and some breast cancer survivors seem to grow from the experience (Brandão et al., 2017). Resilience, which refers to the behaviors, thoughts, and actions that enable persons to adapt to stressful experiences, is a trait that leads to favorable adjustment to stressful events such as breast cancer. All persons possess varying levels of resilience. When persons are successful in meeting life's challenges with resilience, they are more likely to meet subsequent challenges with resilience. Further, there is some evidence that indicates resilience leads to neuroplasticity or the brain's ability to rewire and develop (Hunter et al., 2018). Specifically, higher levels of resilience are related to distinct morphological changes in brain regions that are associated with executive functioning and emotional arousal networks (Gupta et al., 2017).

While resilience relates to adaptation to stressful events, resilience does not necessarily result in psychological growth. Posttraumatic growth, however, involves psychologically moving beyond pre-trauma levels of adjustment (Mohr & Rosen, 2017). Posttraumatic growth is defined as favorable psychological alterations a person experiences after a stressful and/or traumatic event (Maitilis, 2020). Not all persons who experience trauma are able to achieve posttraumatic growth. There are several factors that either promote or negate one's capacity to develop posttraumatic growth, such as how persons handle their emotions and respond to their emotions when confronted with trauma (Jayawickreme et al., 2020). Posttraumatic growth not only leads to enhanced psychological wellness in the long term, but it also results in positive alterations in the brain (Kielb et al., 2019). Posttraumatic growth results in neuroplasticity, which involves the ability to make new brain-based connections.

In learning of a breast cancer diagnosis, being confronted with one's own mortality, and enduring aggressive treatment, breast cancer survivors can experience posttraumatic stress. Posttraumatic growth theory suggests that some degree of distress is necessary to stimulate growth (Zebrack et al., 2015). In the long term, however, breast cancer survivors are credited with being resilient following this experience, and at times, breast cancer survivors may grow as a result of the emotional experiences and conditions they endured. Most breast cancer survivors appreciate long-term healthy adjustment, but others seem to flourish beyond this (Brandão et al., 2017). The majority of breast cancer survivors view their cancer experience as more positive than negative; however, a minority of survivors achieve posttraumatic growth (McDonough et al., 2014). Many survivors report psychological growth because they feel stronger for withstanding treatment, while also feeling gratitude for surviving a life-compromising physical condition (Loeffler et al., 2018). When breast cancer survivors experience enhanced psychological wellbeing following treatment, this is referred to as posttraumatic growth. Maintaining resilience during the course of treatment has been positively linked to posttraumatic growth (Leung et al., 2014). At the same time, cancer patients who endorsed a moderate level of lifetime stress reported a greater degree of posttraumatic growth in the long term (Dooley et al., 2017).

There are multiple individual factors that can influence one's capacity for growth and resilience, one of them being early life physical and/or emotional abuse. One aspect of emotional abuse is best described by John Bowlby's attachment theory, which determined that multiple disruptions in relationships with primary caregivers lead to greater delinquency, increased depression, aggression, and undesirable characterological traits. These insecure attachments of early childhood, when persistent and severe, have been associated with psychopathology in adulthood (Bretherton, 1992). While many studies explore factors, such as social support, that can contribute to this growth following breast cancer, this study examines earlier life experiences that can facilitate some women's achieving posttraumatic growth. Specifically, this study explores whether women who have experienced childhood abuse may develop resilience to further life vicissitudes and after breast cancer may be able to achieve posttraumatic growth.

The literature is laden with studies that examined psychopathology associated with childhood abuse (Adams et al., 2018). There is limited information as to whether persons with a history of abuse are able to develop some type of strength in response to abuse and whether this strength helps them in growing when confronted with future challenges. Two types of such mental fortitude are resilience and posttraumatic growth. Although resilience and posttraumatic growth are both associated with mental toughness, these constructs are quite different. Resilience connotes maintaining psychological wellbeing when confronted with tragedy, while posttraumatic growth refers to positive changes that result from working through tragedy (Tedeschi & Calhoun, 2004). In other words, when persons are resilient, they utilize innate traits to overcome obstacles. Such resilience may help persons better cope while dealing with distress, but there is no necessary long-term impact of resilience. With posttraumatic growth, persons are impacted by trauma. When such persons are able to transcend such trauma, this leads to long-term posttraumatic growth, which suggests they are better from the experience. It is possible that resilience and posttraumatic growth determined from adverse experiences in childhood may help such persons develop mental fortitude in meeting subsequent challenges.

While there is a wealth of literature that focuses on the undesirable impact of early-life abuse, exploration of whether adverse childhood experiences can lead to personal growth is limited (Schaefer et al., 2018). The ill effects of childhood adverse experiences that involve internalized and externalized psychopathology may lead to low resilience. In contrast, Mohr and Rosén (2017) found that university students with a history of adverse events in childhood were more likely to have experienced both posttraumatic stress disorder and posttraumatic growth as compared to those with no such history. When persons are able to develop resilience in response to childhood abuse, this enhances posttraumatic growth (Tranter et al., 2020). Based upon literature reviewed, persons who experience some form of trauma, such as abuse, may exhibit greater degrees of posttraumatic growth when faced with future challenges such as breast cancer. What has not been explored is whether resilience achieved in response to abusive experiences in childhood helps women achieve posttraumatic growth when confronted with stressful events in adulthood, such as breast cancer diagnosis and treatment.

Posttraumatic growth theory posits that persons may also determine mental fortitude in response to such adverse events. In turn, the strength due to some adverse events in childhood may help promote further growth when these persons are confronted with traumatic events during adulthood. One of the struggles persons may potentially confront in adulthood is breast cancer. In fact, persons with a history of childhood abuse are at greater risk for developing cancer in adulthood, as compared to those with no abuse history (Hovdestad et al., 2020). From the moment of diagnosis, women tend to experience immediate anxiety due to potential loss of life, as well as fear of the harsh treatment that lies ahead (Brandão et al., 2017). When treatment is initiated, anxiety intensifies, and depression may begin. Adjustment issues associated with the rigors of treatment involve alterations in body image, physical and mental fatigue, and pain associated with surgery and therapeutic interventions (Bellizzi & Blank, 2006). While diagnosis and treatment tend to be traumatic in nature, in the long term, breast cancer survivors often report resiliency and posttraumatic growth for withstanding the harsh treatment, and for surviving a life-compromising physical ailment (Loeffler et al., 2018).

Although experiences of abuse during childhood have been linked with increased psychopathology in adulthood, a moderate level of lifetime stress has been associated with greater resilience (Dooley et al., 2017). Because persons with low levels of lifetime stress endorse less resilience, this supports the notion that experience in working through previous hardships may cause persons to be better equipped to work successfully through subsequent difficulties, such as breast cancer. Conversely, Dooley et al. (2017) further suggest that persons with a history of severe distress may feel overwhelmed to the extent that they cannot establish a fortifying effect, such as with a history of moderate lifetime stress. Due to the range in outcomes from lifetime stress, when exploring resilience and posttraumatic growth in breast cancer survivors, it is important to contemplate the severity of abuse. Thus, the aim of this study is to examine the impact that childhood physical and emotional abuse, as well as the degrees of abuse severity, have on resilience and posttraumatic growth among breast cancer survivors.

Past scholars have primarily focused on the negative effects of adverse experiences in childhood. There has been no examination as to whether resilience determined from abusive experiences in childhood helps persons in meeting adulthood challenges with resilience, such as breast cancer. For instance, Guil et al. (2020) focused on factors that contribute to resilience in breast cancer survivors such as social support and spirituality, without taking into consideration the survivors' life experiences. The current study will fill a gap in the literature regarding a lack of research and knowledge on how adverse childhood experiences affect breast cancer survivors' resiliency and posttraumatic growth. The aim of this study is to offer insight into therapeutic techniques that may assist women in manifesting resiliency after confronting the challenges of breast cancer treatment.

CHAPTER TWO: REVIEW OF THE LITERATURE

This study investigates whether breast cancer survivors with a history of adverse experiences during childhood show greater levels of perceived posttraumatic growth and resilience as compared to those who have not experienced adverse childhoods. Multiple scholars have investigated the negative effects and consequences of childhood trauma, but they have not fully examined whether some adverse experiences may also stimulate growth (Schaefer et al., 2018). In line with this observation, this study investigates the development of resilience and experiences of posttraumatic growth of breast cancer survivors with a history of adverse childhood experiences.

This chapter will provide an overview of breast cancer statistics as related to occurrence and mortality. Breast cancer staging, common forms of treatment, and stages of survival will also be reviewed. This chapter ventures to explain the psychological adjustment and anxiety-related trauma breast cancer survivors may experience at the time of diagnosis, during treatment, and following treatment conclusion. Next, the concept of resilience, which is associated with favorable adaptation to traumatic events, will be explored in relation to breast cancer survival. Following that, the construct of posttraumatic growth, which is the capacity to develop psychological growth in response to traumatic events, such as breast cancer, will be discussed. Additionally, the literature review will examine whether certain types of early-life experiences, such as childhood abuse, will enhance a woman's capacity to meet the diagnosis of and treatment for breast cancer with resilience, and subsequently develop posttraumatic growth. This chapter presents an extensive review of the studies that examine resiliency and posttraumatic growth of persons with a history of childhood abuse as well as resiliency and posttraumatic growth of breast cancer survivors. I reviewed studies that supported the gap in the research and what previous scholars did to address the problem and their recommendations. A discussion on the theoretical framework underpinning the study will be offered. After a chapter summary, current literature supporting the identified problem will be provided as a culmination of the literature review section.

Breast Cancer

According to the American Cancer Society *Facts and Figures Report* (2022) an estimated 43,780 breast cancer deaths (43,250 in women, 530 in men) will occur in 2022 (Islami et al, 2022). Breast cancer is the second highest cause of cancer death in women, second to lung cancer. Breast cancer accounts for a third of the cancer incidence in women and a quarter of the total cancer incidence. Due to an increase in early detection, which enhances the opportunity for survival, there are more than 3.8 million breast cancer survivors in the United States (Islami et al, 2022).

Breast Cancer Stages

After the initial distress of the breast cancer diagnosis, anxiety often intensifies as treatment planning begins. Cancer staging is then completed to outline appropriate treatment. Generally, physicians use diagnostic imaging and biopsies to assess 1- (T) the tumor size and its biomarkers; 2- (N) whether cancer has left the breast and spread to nodes within the lymph system; and 3- (M) whether cancer spread from the lymph system to other parts of the body (Greene & Kosinski, 2018). The tumor is classified within 1 of 5 stages. The lower the stage, the greater likelihood of survival. No evidence of a tumor marks T_0. With T_1, the tumor size is 20 mm or smaller. For T_3, the tumor is larger than 50 mm. T_4 is determined by one of the following: 1- T_4a: the tumor has grown into the chest wall; 2- T_4b: the tumor has grown into the skin; 3-T_4c: the tumor has grown into the chest wall and the skin; or 4- T_4d: the presence of inflammatory breast cancer, which is a rare and aggressive disease in which cancer cells block lymph vessels in the skin of the breast (Giuliano et al., 2018). Lymph node classification is as follows: 1- N_0: no positive nodes; 2- N_1: 4 to 9 positive nodes; 3- N_3: 10 or more positive lymph nodes. Metastasis classification includes 1- M_x: metastasis cannot be determined; 2- M_0: no evidence of metastasis; 3- M_0 (i+): no metastasis revealed on imaging, but there is microscopic evidence of tumor cells in the blood, marrow, or lymph nodes; 4- M_1; breast cancer cells are found and are growing in one or more organs of the body (Greene & Kosinski, 2018).

Breast Cancer Treatment

Generally, advanced cancer is treated more aggressively than tumors diagnosed at earlier stages (Waks & Winer, 2019). For instance, for a patient with Stage 1 cancer, treatment may be limited to a lumpectomy, which involves removing the tumor and tissue in the surrounding area in conjunction with radiation. Surgery recovery lasts only a few weeks. Radiation treatment occurs five times per week for several weeks, and side effects are mild in most cases, such as burning of the skin and generalized fatigue. Beyond Stage 1, there is an increased need for mastectomy/breast removal of one or both breasts (Trayes & Cokenakes, 2021). Recuperation lasts 6 weeks. Some women may choose to have breast implants, which entails several plastic surgery visits, and at least one additional surgery. Stage 2 and more advanced cases often require adjunctive chemotherapy. Factors that impact chemo dosing involve the age of the patient, as well as disease progression. For instance, a 31-year-old patient with Stage 3-C cancer will receive a higher dose of chemotherapy versus an 80-year-old with Stage 2-B breast cancer (Chan & Abd Hamid, 2021).

Common complications associated with the three most common intravenous chemotherapy medicines include nausea, vomiting, dehydration, headaches, fever, hot flashes, fatigue, and hair loss (Trayes & Cokenakes, 2021). Less common yet more problematic side effects include sepsis, Clostridioides difficile (C-diff), thrush, kidney damage, and sometimes death if patients do not receive emergency care when needed. Some breast cancer patients are maintained on long-term oral medications when tumors are identified as being hormone receptor-positive/fueled by hormones (Waks & Winer, 2019). Side effects are less severe than chemotherapy, but symptoms persist throughout treatment, which lasts a few years. These side effects can include fatigue, low libido, dry mouth, and malaise.

The positive diagnosis of breast cancer is often a shock for most women, because most persons are asymptomatic at the time of diagnosis. It is common for newly diagnosed persons to primarily be concerned with the basic need for survival instead of higher-level matters, such as alteration in body image (Hill & Watkins, 2017). Thus, women tend to be highly motivated for treatment, while they tend to experience anxiety regarding treatment decision making, such as the type of surgery. Prior to treatment survivors are often fearful regarding surgical removal of their breasts and chemotherapy, which can cause temporary loss of hair. In particular, the anxiety about the desire to survive, as well as one's mortality, both are a source of anxiety. As treatment progresses, and cancer patients become more confident in their potential for survival, they tend to struggle with body image issues (Grogan & Mechan, 2017). Following a mastectomy and possible weight changes during chemotherapy, they face body image issues marked by a lack of self-confidence and increased self-consciousness. Women are often betrayed by their bodies, and they experience sexual side effects due to low estrogen and chemically induced menopause. Following mastectomy and reconstruction, women often are dissatisfied with their appearance and they also lose breast sensation (Chan & Abd Hamid, 2021). Problems with sexual intimacy are common, particularly due to the preceding issues related to breast loss, unmet expectations with reconstruction and breast cosmesis, weight gain, hair loss, and menopausal treatment effects that include vulvovaginal changes (e.g., dryness, dyspareunia). For this reason, breast cancer patients and survivors often benefit from a comprehensive oncological program, which in addition to crucial medical care involves participation in support groups and individual psychotherapy (Swainston et al., 2020).

Stages of Survival

When harsh treatment concludes, some level of anxiety may continue as women worry as to whether they will survive in the long term (i.e., fear of recurrence). The 5-year survival rate for breast cancer is more than 85% with less than 15% of cases being classified as Stage 3-4, which are locally advanced or metastatic (Gathani et al., 2021). The death rate associated with breast cancer has steadily declined over the past several decades (Niakan et al., 2021). Since 2001, there has been a steady decline in the 5-year mortality rate. In 2020, 1 in 8 diagnosed with breast cancer died, which is an improvement from the 2001 statistics that reflect a 1 in 6 statistic. One reason for the reduced breast cancer mortality is the increased aim at early detection (Marks et al., 2015). Specifically, annual or biannual mammograms, public education, including the need for self-breast exams, and increased breast cancer screenings, have reduced the likelihood of advanced or metastatic disease by 20%. When breast cancer occurs, it is more likely to be diagnosed earlier. Countless studies have indicated that a woman's likelihood of surviving breast cancer sharply increases when diagnosed at Stage 1 or 2 instead of Stage 3 or 4 (Marks et al., 2015). The unfortunate fact is that public health measures aimed at early detection and prevention of breast cancer have been more successful with middle-class and upper-class women than women of lower socioeconomic status. One potential explanation for this population's reluctance in medical care is that they may be reluctant to seek treatment from a healthcare system that may have failed them in the past (Marks et al., 2015).

Cancer survivorship is marked by the number of years living past cancer diagnosis. Often, breast cancer patients are referred to as survivors from the time of diagnosis or minimally at the onset of treatment. Short-term survivorship is classified as living up to 5 years post cancer diagnosis (Rowland, 2007). Historically, the classification of long-term survivorship ranges from 3 to 5 years post initial diagnosis. Due to longer survival periods, long-term survivorship is currently defined as living past the diagnosis of cancer for 5 to 10 years, and persons living beyond 10 years past diagnosis are considered very long-term survivors (Chan & Abd Hamid, 2021).

Psychological Adjustment to Breast Cancer

From the onset of diagnosis, throughout treatment, and following the conclusion of treatment, breast cancer is a highly charged emotional experience. Stanton et al. (2007) describe psychological adjustment to breast cancer as a dynamic process, wherein it is common for patients to experience either clinical or subclinical symptoms of depression and anxiety following diagnosis and during treatment (Brandão et al., 2017). Such adjustment concerns are often associated with rigorous treatments, which cause pain, fatigue, and a host of physical symptoms; fear of loss of life; and potential new-onset or ongoing/unresolved issues with body image. Women may experience high levels of anxiety in the time period after diagnosis, before surgery (Drageset et al., 2010). Women who endorsed lower levels of anxiety during this timeframe tended to suppress emotions, while managing life as usual (Drageset et al., 2010). Emotional suppression in earlier stages of treatment has been shown to be associated with higher levels of anxiety as treatment progresses (Schlatter & Cameron, 2010; Silva et al., 2012).

There is considerable variability in the long-term psychological adjustment of breast cancer survivors. Following conclusion of treatment and over the course of time, some breast cancer survivors continue to experience anxiety and depression, while other women learn to psychologically adjust. Some women think they feel mentally stronger for having endured treatment. Generally, women who initially suffer from anxiety and despair during treatment, but then undergo a positive psychological transformation, tend to have a favorable adjustment in the long term (Silva et al., 2012). There is a common theme for those women who have healthier adjustment. Typically, they experience unsettling emotions in response to breast cancer/treatment, but then they are able to work through the distress. Specifically, long-term adjustment does not occur with breast cancer patients who avoid undesirable emotions (Drageset et al., 2010). Rather, posttraumatic growth is associated with mood deterioration, processing the emotional experience, and subsequently achieving emotional growth. When favorable psychological adjustment is marked by a life-altering mindset and nuanced sense of self and others, this refers to posttraumatic growth.

Breast Cancer and Posttraumatic Stress

Posttraumatic stress is often viewed as the psychological result of a negative, unexpected event or a series of events to which a person is exposed such as combat, an accident, and/or abuse. However, the experience of trauma also can occur due to sudden onset health problems that cause persons to contemplate their own mortality. Since 1994, there has been increased attention to the prevalence and characteristics of cancer-related PTSD (Kangas, 2013). It is common for newly diagnosed patients, as well as patients undergoing treatment, to have symptoms of PTSD. Fearfulness related to loss of life, aggressive treatments that threaten self-integrity, and the intense feelings of helplessness related to a diagnosis and treatment for cancer may occur. Further, because most survivors are asymptomatic at the time of diagnosis, learning of this unexpected, negative event of cancer is anxiety provoking. Based upon DSM-5 criteria, 35% of cancer patients experience anxiety (i.e., an adjustment disorder with anxious mood or PTSD). Specific symptoms of PTSD tend to be those associated with re-experiencing treatment or diagnosis (nightmares or flashbacks), avoidance of reminders of the disease or treatment (denial or numb affect), and hyperarousal (exaggerated startle response, sleep disturbances; Andrykowski et al., 2008). The symptoms of PTSD may be manifested as constant worry, fears of cancer recurrence, nightmares about the illness or treatments, and additional psychological symptoms, such as irritability and anger, which may impact interpersonal relationships negatively (Bush, 2009). Not only do these psychological symptoms cause distress, but they can also negatively impact survival.

Following treatment, one of the most significant sources of anxiety is fear of cancer recurrence. Fang et al. (2018) found that fear of recurrence was the most often reason expressed for anxiety in women who had survived cancer for at least 5 years. There was a positive association with reduced anxiety and years of survival. Although some element of anxiety exists in the long term, it is important to discern whether anxiety is excessive as compared to anxieties people face in general. A study of the health information of 814 very long-term breast cancer survivors, who survived 15 years or more, found that breast cancer survivors had similar levels of anxiety as compared to the general population (Stava et al., 2006). While some may continue to struggle emotionally, many breast cancer survivors overcome cancer-related anxiety in the long term. Long-term survivors of breast cancer generally report good health and quality of life, although 30.4% of breast cancer survivors report that cancer has affected their health and quality of life (Stava et al., 2006).

Many breast cancer survivors, in the long term, learn to adapt. Breast cancer survivors as a whole are credited with possessing mental fortitude, and many report favorable mental health after treatment ends and after treatment effects are over. Considerable attention has been dedicated to examining what causes some persons to languish while others flourish. While lingering physical symptoms have been positively linked to ongoing mental distress, some appear to learn to adapt and experience psychological wellness (Spiegel, 2012). Positive adaptation in the behaviors, thoughts, and actions of women recovering from breast cancer is termed resilience.

Resilience

Meeting various life challenges in general with resilience has been positively associated with favorable mental health in the long term (Dockray & Steptoe, 2010). In this next section, the various definitions of resilience will be discussed. Factors that cause persons to meet challenges with psychological resilience will be reviewed. Additionally, this discussion will entail exploring neuropsychological factors associated with resilience.

Resiliency Defined

A literature review reveals that there is not one universal definition of resilience. Generally, resilience can be described as a favorable result of a multifaceted adaption to adversity and the ability to access and utilize resources when confronted with traumatic events (Schulz et al., 2014). Resiliency is considered a dynamic personality trait that is flexible, allowing persons to react to adversity. Additional definitions of resilience refer to it as a trait often described as the individual's ability to solve problems during stressful situations or traumatic events (Masten et al., 2019). In synthesizing these definitions, it appears that resiliency is comprised of favorable cognitive and emotional responses to tragedy that cause persons to flourish versus experience emotional turmoil.

There are several common traits associated with resiliency. Resilient persons seek social support, take care of themselves, engage in needed recreational activities, and find a balance between rest and responsibility. Positive affect, self-efficacy, optimism, social support, self-esteem, and life satisfaction have been more highly associated with resilience than sociodemographic factors, such as being raised in poverty versus prosperity (Martínez-Martí & Ruch, 2017). Positive affect relates to experiencing positive emotions and expression. Positive affect has been associated with positive health outcomes, and it is likely that several biological processes mediate the effects of positive mood on physical health (Dockray & Steptoe, 2010). Therefore, resilience not only is a means of maintaining positive mood while confronting the challenges of breast cancer, but it also may contribute to physical wellbeing. For instance, Peterson et al. (2006) as cited in Martínez-Martí & Ruch (2017) observed that individuals who had recovered from a physical illness or a psychological disorder scored higher in some character strengths than individuals without such a history. Following physical illness, those who endorsed resiliency reported greater bravery, kindness, and humor. The most significant association with physical illness and resiliency was bravery, which suggests that stronger levels of bravery can be useful to these same persons when working through subsequent challenges. Appreciation of beauty and love of learning mediated the association between a history of psychological disorder and greater life satisfaction after recovery. Capacity for resilience is developed as a result of genetics, temperament, and environment.

A review of the literature reveals that resilience is often referred to as either a trait or a state. Resilience as a trait refers to generally inherent characteristics, strengths, or aspects of temperament, which are stable over time (Kuldas & Foody, 2022). As a state, resilience refers to cognitions and emotions that are malleable and can be strengthened with adaptation. In this sense, state resilience is described as an outcome, whereas trait resilience is considered a constant (Jones, 2002). From a transactional perspective, resilience is considered both a trait and a state. With this integrated conceptualization, resilience is a developmental process, capacity, and outcome despite adverse life events. It is a dynamic process that involves evolution within the individual, and it enables positive adaptation in response to adversity (Kuldas & Foody, 2022).

One of the most striking examples of resiliency is Viktor Frankl, a psychiatrist who was maintained prisoner in a concentration camp in Nazi Germany. When confronted with the pain, fear, isolation, and hunger associated with his imprisonment, he attempted to derive meaning in life. He realized that he had to find some purpose in his experience. He visualized himself offering lectures after the war in regard to finding meaning in response to trauma. Following his release, to assist others in determining their resiliency, he wrote, "But there was no need to be ashamed of tears, for tears bore witness that a man had the greatest of courage, the courage to suffer" (Frankl, 1985, p. 101). Frankl clearly possessed trait resilience, but he also manifested state resilience when confronting his confinement. The premorbid trait resilience enabled him to establish state resilience when confronted with extreme tragedy.

The Predictive 6-Factor Resilience Scale (PR6) is a measure of psychological resilience that assesses resilience based upon the following domains: vision, composure, tenacity, reasoning, collaboration, and momentum (Rossouw & Rossouw, 2016). Vision relates to the ability to engage in self-efficacy and goal setting, which encompasses hopefulness and optimism. Vision is a function of both innate temperament as well as state resilience. Composure is associated with the capacity for emotional regulation, self-control, and self-awareness. Tenacity refers to the ability to persevere with hardiness in order to overcome significant challenges. Reasoning is the aspect of resiliency that is associated with resiliency because it relates to problem-solving, ingenuity, growing through adversity, and continuing to thrive/flourish when confronted with adversity. Reasoning is transactional in nature because it is comprised of crystalized abilities, as well as learning from experience. Collaboration is the quality of psychosocial interaction, including secure attachment, support networks, context, and humor. Momentum relates to approaching problems with a sense of direction and openness to new challenges (Rossouw & Rossouw, 2016).

While the above six characteristics are considered essential aspects of resiliency, Rossouw and Rossouw (2016) included a 7th factor, health hygiene. Health hygiene, the capacity to engage in favorable self-care, facilitates healthy adaption to adversity. Tugade et al. (2004) as cited within Rossouw and Rossouw (2016) indicated an association between emotional experience and health based upon the effect of higher resilience in suppressing autonomic arousal in the hypothalamic-pituitary-adrenal axis. HPA arousal increases cortisol levels which reduces potential for healthy neural adaptation.

Rossouw et al. (2017) studied domain-level validation of the 16-item Predictive 6-Factor Resilience Scale (PR6), while also devising an extended 50-item scale. A multi-stage testing format was used with 617 adult participants, median age 43, who were recruited via online platform, as well as from educational and healthcare settings. As cited within Rossouw et al. (2017), four items were added based upon the four basic needs: Epstein (2003): maximization of pleasure and minimization of pain; Freud (1909): control and orientation, which is the need for a sense of stability predictability, and meaningfulness; Rogers (1951): relatedness, which is the need for stable and secure attachment relationships with others; and Bowlby (2008): self-enhancement is the need to improve the status of the self. Work from Kohut (1971) and Allport (1961) contributes to the concept of personal growth and improvement. From this, domain-level scales were finalized, an extended 50-item resilience scale (PR6-50) was developed, and the 16-item PR6 was revised. Scales for each domain were validated with good internal consistency (> 0.70). The PR6-50 showed high internal consistency (0.9372), while the revised 16-item PR6 showed improved internal consistency (0.8398).

Neuropsychology of Resiliency

Resilience is thought to be comprised of neurobiological, genetic, temperamental, and environmental factors (Simeon et al., 2007). While much of brain development is inherent, there is an increased understanding of the epigenetic factors, such as those from the environment, which can impact brain development. When persons can manifest resiliency in response to adversity, this results in neuroplasticity, or the brain's ability to rewire and develop (Hunter et al., 2018). It is important to note that resilience does not refer to psychological growth in response to adversity. Resilience is not only a function that helps individuals adapt, but resilience itself also adapts over time (Hunter et al., 2018). General resilience can be strengthened when adapting to specific life's challenges.

There is some additional evidence to support neuroplasticity associated with resilience. Gupta et al. (2017) studied associations between regional brain morphology and trait resilience with a focus on resilience-related morphological differences in brain regions involved in cortico-limbic inhibition. Forty-eight healthy subjects completed structural MRI scans. Subjective, self-reported resilience was measured using the Connor and Davidson Resilience Scale (2003), which is comprised of the following five subscales: 1-self-efficacy, high standards, and tenacity; 2-

emotional and cognitive control under pressure, trust in one's intuition; 3- adaptability/ability to bounce back; 4- sense of control of one's life; 5-faith (Gupta et al., 2017). The Positive Affect Negative Affect (PANAS; Watson et al., 1998) was used to measure both positive affect (e.g., attentive, interested, alert, excited, enthusiastic, inspired, proud, determined, strong, and active) and negative affect (e.g., distressed, upset-distressed, hostile, irritable-angry, scared, afraid-fearful, ashamed, guilty, nervous, and jittery). Findings showed subjective measures of resilience were significantly associated with morphological changes in subregions of the parietal cortex, cingulate subregions, and in the amygdala. Findings also showed a significant, positive morphological association in the executive control network with self-reported resiliency. Self-report measures of resilience were positively associated with positive affect, and negatively associated with negative affect (Gupta et al., 2017). The results of this study suggest that there are neuropsychological factors that contribute to resilience. Specifically, higher levels of resilience are related to distinct morphological alterations in brain regions involved in executive control and emotional arousal networks. The neuropsychological indices suggest that there is an association between trait resilience and affect.

In comparing fMRI findings of adolescents with a history of child maltreatment Galinowski et al. (2015) found fractional anisotropy (FA) in corpus callosum segments II and III in resilient subjects as compared to adolescents who did endorse resilience (Teicher & Samson, 2016). They also observed a linear trend for corpus callosal activity to be greater in resilient subjects than controls, and greater in controls than susceptible subjects. Additionally, an fMRI study of altered autobiographical memory (ABM) processing evaluated potential developmental plasticity in neural functioning following maltreatment (Puetz et al., 2021). The study was comprised of 37 adolescents, 19 with a documented history of maltreatment, and 18 without a history of documented childhood maltreatment. Subjects were monitored fMRI on recalled specific ABMs in response to emotionally triggering cue words. Psychological assessments were collected at both timepoints. Longitudinal analyses were carried out with BOLD signal changes during ABM recall and psychopathology to investigate change over time. In both groups there was relative stability of the ABM brain network, with some developmental maturational changes. Significantly increased activation of the right retrosplenial cortex was observed only in the MT group, which was associated with improved psychological functioning. The authors conclude that this study provides evidence of functional developmental plasticity in children with documented maltreatment.

Resilience and Breast Cancer

As discussed earlier, transactional resilience is an innate as well as developed construct that is employed during times of struggle in order for persons to adapt to adverse circumstances. Resilience involves both adaptation as well as hardening. Di Giacomo et al. (2016) examined psychological resilience in young women (ages 31 to 51), before, during, and after breast cancer treatment. The sample comprised 82 women, 42 of whom were diagnosed with breast cancer and 40 were healthy controls. The goal of the study was to analyze emotional distress of the breast cancer sample with regard to depression, anxiety, and psychological distress. Participants were administered the Psychological Distress Inventory, State-Trait Expression Inventory-2, State-Trait Anxiety Inventory, and the Beck Depression Inventory-II. Psychological resilience was determined indirectly based upon the results of the preceding measures. A one-way ANOVA showed no significant difference between breast cancer and non-breast cancer groups in anger and anxiety factors; in the depression variable, the cancer group was significantly different than the control group, $F(1,79) = 6.63$; $p<.001$. Results revealed that, although they endorsed feeling more anxious and depressed as compared to their pre-diagnosis state, breast cancer patients showed no signs of a new-onset mood disorder. The MANOVA analysis comparing types of psychological distress at various phases of treatment (following diagnosis, status post-surgery, following chemotherapy, and during follow-up hormone treatment) indicated that breast cancer patients' level of resiliency remained relatively the same. This study did not explore factors such as adverse experiences in childhood, which could potentially affect resiliency or contribute to posttraumatic growth (Di Giacomo et al., 2016).

Persons who experience minimal adversity are not challenged to learn to adapt to challenging circumstances. Conversely, persons who experience multiple life stressors learn to adapt when resilient. Because resilience relates to both adaption as well as hardening, some studies have examined whether the effects of favorable emotional responses are long-lasting. Guil et al. (2020) analyzed the differences in emotional intelligence and resilience between breast cancer survivors versus those with no breast cancer history. The hypothesis was that women with a breast cancer history would experience a higher degree of both emotional intelligence and greater resilience. The authors also hypothesized that perceived emotional intelligence, marked by emotional attention, clarity, and repair, can mediate the relationship between breast cancer and resilience. Although the authors used the standard working definition of resilience, in that resilience is a means of adaptation, they theorized that resilience is further strengthened when successfully adapting to challenges. Subjects were recruited via random selection through oncology units in Spain. The sample comprised 167 women, 46.7% of whom were breast cancer survivors and 53.3% were healthy controls, with age ranging from 18 to 69 years. In assessing the ability to confront adverse situations, participants completed the Spanish version of the Young Resilience Scale (Wagnild & Young, 1993), the Spanish version of the

Trait Meta-Mood Scale (Salovey et al., 1995), and the Spanish version of a measure of self-perception of emotional competency. Results suggested that breast cancer survivors showed greater resilience and mood repair levels than the control group. Comparison in variables by groups, the ANOVA indicated statistically significant differences in age, resilience, and mood repair, showing that breast cancer women exhibited greater levels of these variables, with a high effect size. Pearson's correlations indicated positive associations between breast cancer survivorship with age, resilience, and mood repair. Besides, resilience was found to be positively related to emotional clarity and mood repair. Age was significantly and positively related to resilience and negatively associated with emotional attention (Guil et al., 2020).

The mediation analysis revealed that the perceived emotional intelligence of breast cancer survivors predicted 28% of the variance of resilience. The authors posited that the direct effects indicated that emotional clarity and mood repair increased resilience levels. Although breast cancer did not predict resilience directly as hypothesized by the authors, this finding is consistent with common working definitions of resilience in that general resilience is a stable trait (Guil et al., 2020). Although this study described positive outcomes associated with breast cancer survivorship, it did not explore preexisting factors, such as adverse experiences in childhood that may impact resilience and posttraumatic growth.

Posttraumatic Growth

In addition to defining posttraumatic growth, an important distinction will be made between resilience and posttraumatic growth. Factors that either enable or inhibit posttraumatic growth will also be reviewed. Additionally, the positive neuropsychological outcomes associated with posttraumatic growth will be discussed.

Posttraumatic Growth Defined

While resilience relates to adapting to adversity, posttraumatic growth refers to the psychological moving beyond pre-trauma levels of adaptation (Mohr & Rosén, 2017). Posttraumatic growth (PTG) is defined as the positive psychological changes that one experiences after a stressful or traumatic event (Maitlis, 2020). Posttraumatic growth describes the ability of individuals involved in traumatic environments to develop positive changes or show positive developments rather than the usual negative health impacts, including posttraumatic stress disorder, depression, and sustained anxiety (Tedeschi & Calhoun, 1995). While PTG does not exclude the negative effects of traumatic experiences, Tedeschi et al. (2018) opined that PTG does allow individuals to perceive and act upon the positive opportunities that the traumatic event brought for growth.

Not all persons who experience trauma are able to achieve posttraumatic growth. There are several factors that are associated with one's capacity to grow beyond the trauma. Emotional, physical, and mental struggles individuals experience during stressful situations dictate whether posttraumatic growth occurs (Infurna & Jayawickreme, 2019). How individuals handle their emotions and respond to such emotions activated by traumatic events impact the long-term outcome of the stressful situations and whether they are able to achieve growth (Jayawickreme et al., 2020). Resilience, as discussed above, is associated with positive affect and emotional control. Because the adaptive handling of emotions promotes a sense of wellbeing, it is possible that higher degrees of resilience may promote posttraumatic growth when confronted with trauma.

Although one may continue to experience some negative emotions associated with the initial trauma, there is an opportunity for positive growth for some persons to develop psychologically in some areas as compared to prior to being exposed to the traumatic event. Posttraumatic growth is the positive changes that come from emotional turmoil, entails a renewed appreciation for life, a nuanced philosophy, and improved interpersonal relationships (Tranter et al., 2020). To achieve posttraumatic growth, one must struggle with posttraumatic stress to overcome the human responses to unexpected negative events. While resilience is a personal attribute that enables persons to handle stress and return to previous level of functioning, posttraumatic growth marks a transformational process due to personal struggles. In making an important distinction between resilience and posttraumatic growth, resilience is measured based upon the following factors: the ability to engage in self-efficacy and establish goals, the capacity for emotional regulation, perseverance/hardiness, problem solving/ingenuity, the ability to collaborate with others and maintain close relationships, self-direction, and favorable health practices (Rossouw & Rossouw, 2016). Posttraumatic growth is measured as a transformational process following a traumatic event that entails growth in the following domains: appreciation of life, relationships with others, new possibilities in life, personal strength, and spiritual change (Tedeschi & Calhoun, 1996). While the characteristics associated with resilience help persons emotionally work through traumatic events, posttraumatic growth is marked by favorable psychological growth in response to a traumatic event.

Neuropsychology of Posttraumatic Growth

While the severity of trauma impacts the extent to which persons are able to derive posttraumatic growth, there are other potential factors that may either impede or enhance the capacity for growth. Specifically, there is an increased understanding that posttraumatic growth yields favorable brain-based changes. Brain-based alterations promote psychological well-being, which may assist persons in meeting subsequent challenges (Kiełb et al., 2019). Posttraumatic growth not only results in neuroplasticity, but posttraumatic growth also results in neurointegration. While neuroplasticity involves the ability to change by making new brain-based connections, neurointegration relates to the ability to integrate those changes and to produce novel interpretations and new meanings in response to the traumatic event. Neurointegration is thought to occur in both the conscious and unconscious mind. Psychotherapy, storytelling, or expressing one's feelings to a friend tend to cultivate neurointegration (Rozentsvit, 2016).

When the notion of posttraumatic growth was investigated initially, neuroplasticity only existed in theory, without empirical evidence. With advances in neuroimaging there is increased evidence for posttraumatic growth resulting in brain growth. Anders et al. (2015) examined neural correlates of PTG in 106 veterans with a primary diagnosis of PTSD and 193 veteran controls with no known PTSD history. Magnetoencephalography (MEG; Hämäläinen & Hari, 2002), which maps brain activity by recording magnetic fields that naturally occur in the brain, was used as the neuroimaging technique. PTSD was assessed using the Clinician-Administered PTSD Scale for DSM-IV-TR (CAPS; Blake et al., 1995) or the Structured Clinical Interview for DSM-IV-TR (SCID; First et al., 2002). PTG was assessed using the Posttraumatic Growth Inventory (PTGI; Tedeschi & Calhoun, 1996). The Deployment Risk and Resilience Inventory (DRRI; King et al., 2006) assessed lifetime trauma exposure pre-deployment, deployment, and post-deployment (Anders et al., 2015).

Results revealed there were no statistically significant differences in the PTG scores between the control group and the PTSD group (Anders et al., 2015). In contrast, the amount of growth per trauma was significantly higher in the control group as compared to the PTSD group. Analysis of the DRRI and the PTGI revealed that control subjects reported more growth per trauma than did PTSD subjects, $p < .001$. In the control group, global synchronous neural interactions (GSNI) decreased significantly with increasing PTG score. Decreased GSNI indicates increased connectivity. The strongest effect was in the medial prefrontal cortex, where it was much stronger and more extensive in the control group than in the PTSD group. Age, gender, and lifetime trauma did not have a statistically significant effect in either group. Anders et al. (2015) concluded that the controls experienced more positive benefit from trauma than the PTSD group due to neural network decorrelation. Specifically, cognitive processing and restructuring that occur after trauma lead to alterations in an individual's belief structure of the world, allowing for the integration of the traumatic event. The implications of the findings of Anders et al. (2015) are that when persons are successfully able to transcend traumatic experiences, such resolution not only results in posttraumatic growth, but it also results in neuroplasticity.

Theoretical Framework

The current study utilizes a posttraumatic growth theory (PTG) theoretical framework. Posttraumatic growth theory was developed and coined by Richard Tedeschi and Lawrence Calhoun, to explain the transformative power of trauma, given that many individuals who experience significant distress seem to experience positive growth (Tedeschi & Calhoun, 1995). Tedeschi et al. (2018) defined posttraumatic growth as the development or experiences of positive psychological changes and development following a stressful situation.

The posttraumatic growth theory was developed to understand how individuals who had experienced trauma or stressful situations achieved growth. To measure these levels of growth, Tedeschi and Calhoun (1996) developed a posttraumatic growth theory inventory that examined five key positive responses in people who have overcome traumatic situations. The first positive response was personal strength, which is described as an increased feeling of self-reliance, acceptance of outcomes in life, ability to handle difficulties or challenges, and awareness of their new mental strength (Tedeschi & Calhoun, 1996). Personal strength characterizes optimism and self-determination, key tenets of positive psychology. The second positive response is spiritual change. In their earlier studies on posttraumatic growth, Tedeschi and Calhoun (2004) asserted that for decades, different forms of religion tried to explain the renewed sense of living that was projected by individuals who had been through difficult, traumatic situations. As a form of positive psychological growth, the spiritual change described an advanced understanding of spiritual matters and an increased reliance on matters of faith.

The third positive aspect of PTG theory was described by new possibilities that Tedeschi et al. (2018) described as the individual's development of new interests, engagement in productive activities, new opportunities for growth, and an intense need to experience positive change. Linked to psychological characteristics, Tedeschi et al. (2018) equated the aspect of new possibilities to finding meaning and purpose in life. The fourth positive change was relating to others, which described an individual's increased relationship with others in times of difficulty, compassion and friendship for others in difficult situations, willingness to show and express emotions, and development of increased care for others. The fifth and last aspect of PTG is a renewed appreciation for life, which Tedeschi et al. (2018) described as increased value for life, daily appreciation for life, and increased value for things that matter in life.

A method of understanding posttraumatic growth following childhood maltreatment is to explore adults' retrospective recall of abuse and the impact on growth (Reuben et al., 2016). Jankovic et al. (2022) examined the relationship between a history of child maltreatment (HCM) and well-being among young adults in relation to both the severity of the maltreatment, as well as posttraumatic growth (PTG). Participants consisted of 537 young adults (aged 18–25; M = 21.09) from across Australia, with 182 young adults in the sample forming the cohort with a HCM. Participants' current well-being, the extent of maltreatment by their mother, father, and other adults experienced as a child (<18 years), and PTG was collected using an online survey. The overall well-being subscale of the Positive Emotions, Engagement, Relationships, Meaning, and Accomplishment (PERMA) Profiler was used to measure current well-being. It includes 15 items measuring the dimensions, and one happiness item (Butler & Kern, 2016). The 22-item Comprehensive Child Maltreatment Scale (CCMS) (Higgins & McCabe, 2001) measured self-reported child maltreatment experiences before age 18. Respondents rated how frequently they witnessed family violence, or endured neglect, sexual abuse, physical abuse, and psychological abuse behavior by their mother, father, or other adults. After having completed the child maltreatment questions, participants subjectively indicated if they thought that they had experienced child maltreatment by responding "yes" (n = 112) or "maybe" (n = 88). Those who endorsed a history of maltreatment based upon the rating scale or based upon subjective recall were as having a history of child maltreated. Those with a history of child maltreatment completed the Posttraumatic Growth Inventory (PTGI; Tedeschi & Calhoun, 1996) in relation to their experiences of child maltreatment. Participants who responded "no" (n = 337) skipped the PTGI and were debriefed at the end of the survey. Tests of group differences and multiple regression were conducted to analyze the relationships between child maltreatment, PTG, and current well-being. Young adults who identified as having a HCM had poorer well-being than those who did not. Within the cohort of those with a HCM, greater PTG predicted greater well-being, and also mitigated the negative relationship between child maltreatment by one's father and well-being. The authors concluded that PTG played a protective role, which suggested the potential therapeutic benefit of fostering PTG to improve well-being among young adults with a HCM (Jankovic et al., 2022). Although this study highlighted the association between PTG in relation to psychological wellbeing, following HCM, the study did not explore the extent to which PTG helps persons deal with life challenges in adulthood.

There is increased evidence that some persons are able to achieve elements of growth in response to traumatic events throughout the lifespan. Wu et al. (2019) completed a systematic meta-analytic review of 26 studies on posttraumatic stress disorder and posttraumatic growth, which specifically analyzed physical and emotional trauma in adults. The analysis was completed by placing the type of trauma into one of three different categories: disease, accident, and specific profession. Specific profession refers to firefighters, veterans, intensive care staff, and so on. Results indicated that 52.58% of people who had experienced traumatic events showed moderate to high PTG, which buffered them against depression, anxiety, and stress. Similar results were presented by Slade et al. (2019), who conducted quantitative research with 77 participants with mental health challenges following a traumatic event and found that 83% reported PTG described by increased spirituality, appreciation for life, personal strength, and a renewed sense of purpose, and overcome burnout, emotional exhaustion, and trauma through teamwork and personal strength.

According to Tedeschi and Calhoun (2004), at least 89% of stressful and traumatic situations survivors reported experiencing some form of posttraumatic growth, such as a renewed appreciation for life. At the same time, it was expected that experiences of negative trauma(s) more often resulted in negative growth characterized by conditions such as posttraumatic stress disorder and other significant mental health disorders, including depression and long-term experiences of an anxiety disorder (Tedeschi et al., 2018). In fact, a meta-analytic review of 14 studies on the negative long-term consequences of childhood abuse revealed that these children are at greater risk of developing depression in adulthood (Carr et al., 2020). In examining the positive side of experiencing trauma, Tedeschi et al. (2018) established that rather than developing adverse mental health conditions, the traumatic experiences triggered the development of transformative personality in certain individuals.

Because some persons develop posttraumatic growth in response to trauma, while others do not, it is important to understand conditions that may either yield or detract from PTG. Calhoun et al. (2000) examined factors that can impact posttraumatic growth, such as the degree to which event-related rumination, a quest orientation to religion, and religious involvement are related to posttraumatic growth. Participants consisted of 54 students who had experienced a major traumatic event, 35 women and 19 men, with a mean age of 22.5 years. As cited by Calhoun et al. (2000), the Traumatic Stress Schedule (Norris, 1990) was used to screen for events severe enough to place subjects at risk for posttraumatic stress disorder. As cited by Calhoun et al. (2000), the Quest Scale (Batson et al., 1993) was used to measure religiosity, specifically openness to change, self-criticism, and perception of religious doubt as positive, and readiness to face existential questions without reducing their complexity. Rumination related to the traumatic event was measured by using items from several other instruments developed to assess various aspects of posttraumatic cognitive processing. As cited by Calhoun et al. (2000), religious participation was measured by three items (Wuthnow, 1994) asking whether the respondent was currently attending religious services, how often they attend religious services, and how important religion was in their lives. The Posttraumatic Growth Inventory (PTGI; Tedeschi & Calhoun, 1996), is a 21-item scale that measures the degree of reported positive changes experienced in the struggle with major life crises. The two main factors associated with posttraumatic growth were the degree of self-reported rumination soon after the event (beta = .47), and the degree of openness to religious change (beta = .29). In contrast, ruminations that were intrusive, negative, and persistent led to low levels of growth and high levels of distress.

Construct validity of the PTGI was established by examining the extent to which this assessment measures benefits to trauma (Taku et al., 2008). Specifically, in comparing persons who had experienced trauma to those that had no such history, persons who had experienced severe trauma had higher scores on the New Possibilities factor, F(l,113) = 6.54, $p < .05$, the Relating to Others factor, F{l,113) = 4.95, $p < .05$, the Personal Strength factor, F(l,113) = 9.23, $p < .01$, and the Appreciation of Life factor, F{l,113) = 17.58, $p < .001$, but not the Spiritual Change factor, F(l,113) = 1.12, n.s. The authors suggest that mean scores indicate that persons experiencing severe trauma tend to report a higher degree of change, while persons reporting no extraordinary events report a "small" to "moderate" degree of change. This may indicate that an event that is so extreme as to negate fundamental assumptions may produce more positive change than less challenging circumstances. This affirmed the hypothesis that persons experiencing severe trauma would report more benefit than those who were not confronted with extraordinary events (Tedeschi & Calhoun, 1996).

The sample consisted of 199 men and 405 women ($N = 604$; Taku et al., 2008). Some participants were administered, in addition to the PTGI, in random order, the NEO Personality Inventory ($n = 325$), the LOT ($n = 449$), the Marlowe-Crowne Social Desirability Scale ($n = 318$), and the Index of Religious Participation ($n = 237$). Participants also completed two 6-point Likert ratings: the positive effect and the negative effect the event had on the person, ranging from "no effect" to "extreme effect." Correlations between the PTGI and other measures mentioned here are at the $p < .01$ or $p < .001$ levels, although others reached significance at $p < .05$ (Taku et al., 2008).

Persons scoring higher on Appreciation of Life reported themselves to be more optimistic and extraverted (Taku et al., 2008). Persons scoring higher on Spiritual Change reported themselves to be more optimistic, religious, and extraverted. Certain specific facets of the major NEO personality domains were primarily responsible for the relationships between those personality factors and the PTGI and its factors. Three facets in particular were related to all PTGI factors and to the total PTGI most strongly: the Extraversion facets of Activity ($r = .31$ with PTGI) and Positive Emotions ($r = .34$ with FI'GI), and the Openness facet of Feelings ($r = .28$ with PTGI). Some specific facets were related to the PTGI factors even though the major domain they comprise were not. For example, the Openness to Experience facet of values was negatively correlated with PTGI Spiritual Change ($r = -.15$). The authors conclude that the NEO personality traits are manifestations of PTGI (Taku et al., 2008).

It is possible to possess elements of both resilience while also developing posttraumatic growth. Tedeschi et al. (2018) defined resiliency as a personal attribute characterized by the ability to bounce back. When described under the lens of PTG, resilience refers to the ability of an individual to return to previous levels of functioning (Tedeschi et al., 2017). After experiencing highly stressful, unexpected, negative situations, some individuals grow and transform positively, which refers to PTG. While the trauma itself does not result in PTG, the changes in cognitive and emotional strength after the incident are what yield growth (Tedeschi et al., 2018).

Resilience as a mediator in the relationship between posttraumatic stress and posttraumatic growth has previously been examined. Lee et al. (2020) examined the moderated mediating effect of childhood trauma on resilience and its associations with posttraumatic stress symptoms (PTSS) and posttraumatic growth (PTG) in adults who were involved in traumatic accidents or crimes. The hypothesis was that resilience would mediate relationships between PTSS and PTG and that its mediating effects would differ depending on childhood trauma. Data were collected from 143 adult participants (mean age = 37.69) in Korea (82 females, 61 males) who were victims of accidents or crimes. To assess PTSD symptoms, 20 items from the PTSD Checklist for DSM-5 (PCL-5) were used (Blevins et al., 2015). Trait resilience was measured using the 25-item Connor-Davidson Resilience Scale (CD-RISC; Connor & Davidson, 2003). The Adverse Childhood Experiences (ACE) questionnaire measured experiences of childhood trauma including physical, emotional, and sexual abuse, as well as violence and neglect (Felitti et al., 1998). Findings indicated that the effect of PTSS on PTG is fully mediated by resilience and that the mediating effect of resilience on the relationship between PTSS and PTG is moderated by childhood trauma levels. Higher levels of childhood trauma were accompanied by greater moderated mediation effects (−1SD = −.0753, mean = −.1138, +1SD = −.1574). The greater the childhood traumatic experiences, the greater the mediating effect of resilience was between PTSS and PTG. The effect of resilience on PTG was greatest in the high childhood trauma group, and high levels of resilience were associated with high levels of PTG regardless of childhood trauma. With lower resilience, however, higher levels of childhood trauma were accompanied by lower levels of PTG, compared to lower levels of childhood trauma. Study results indicate that the mediating effect of resilience can be taken into account in the pathway from PTSS to PTG.

There has been additional research in regard to investigating the mediating role of resiliency between temperamental traits and posttraumatic growth. Data of 74 persons M = 38.4;

SD = 15.5) who have experienced death of someone close were analyzed (Ogińska-Bulik & Kobylarczyk, 2017). The majority of the participants had lost a parent – 37.8%. Among remaining participants: 21.6% had lost a child, 18.9% a spouse or a partner, 10.8% a sibling and 10.8% a very close friend. The Posttraumatic Growth Inventory (PTGI) developed by Tedeschi and Calhoun (1996) was used to assess positive changes in the aftermath of trauma. As cited within Ogińska-Bulik & Kobylarczyk (2017), temperament was assessed by the Formal Characteristics of Behavior Temperament Inventory (FCB-TI) developed by Zawadzki and Strelau (1997), which is comprised of six scales: Briskness, Perseveration, Sensory Sensitivity, Emotional Reactivity, Endurance, and Activity. As cited within Ogińska-Bulik & Kobylarczyk (2017), the Resiliency Assessment Scale by Ogińska-Bulik and Juczyński (2008) was used to measure resiliency based upon 5 factors: (a) Determination and persistence in actions, (b) Openness to new experiences and a sense of humor, (c) Competencies to cope and tolerance of a negative affect, (d) Tolerance of failures and treating life as a challenge, and (e) Optimistic life attitude and ability to mobilize in difficult situations.

Results indicated that resiliency was more strongly associated with PTG following death of a loved one as opposed to temperament (Ogińska-Bulik & Kobylarczyk, 2017). Resiliency positively correlated with PTG, mainly with the PTG traits of changes in self-perception and appreciation of life. The authors concluded that the more significant role of resiliency, compared to temperament, in experiencing positive changes after negative life events indicates that posttraumatic growth is more likely to be determined by skills gained as a result of coping with various difficult situations rather than biological determinants. Therefore, the authors opine that predisposition to experience positive changes in the aftermath of trauma might be harnessed throughout life (Ogińska-Bulik & Kobylarczyk, 2017).

Breast Cancer and Posttraumatic Growth

Although diagnosis and treatment for breast cancer results in anxiety, and sometimes anxiety-related trauma, some women report growth from the experience. Longitudinal studies have assessed psychological adjustment following treatment at some point during survivorship, and some studies, such as Costanzo et al. (2009) and Leung et al. (2014) suggest that most survivors experience healthy adjustment in the long term (Brandão et al., 2017). Some breast cancer survivors not only learn to adjust, but they also grow. Therefore, it is relevant to examine why some breast cancer survivors achieve growth while others do not. In terms of resiliency and posttraumatic growth related to breast cancer survivorship, it is thought that the main contributory factors include the ideation that survivors feel stronger for withstanding harsh treatment and gratitude for surviving a life-compromising physical ailment (Loeffler et al., 2018). Learning of a breast cancer diagnosis and being subjected to treatment can cause perceptions of trauma. Subsequent to treatment, in the long term, when resiliency and posttraumatic growth occur, survivors experience favorable psychological responses to the traumatic event (Brandão et al., 2017).

Positive adaptations can occur following the exposure to traumatic events. These positive adaptations include both resilience and posttraumatic growth. Resilience is a coping strategy that helps trauma survivors recover from the aftereffects of stressors (Loeffler et al., 2018). Posttraumatic growth refers to the positive changes, better adjustments, and positive state of mind in the aftermath of trauma. Breast cancer survivors experience varying degrees of posttraumatic growth. The question is what factors contribute to such growth. Loeffler et al. (2018) reported that resilience and posttraumatic growth played a critical and significant role in promoting breast cancer patients' fight for survival, given their ability to withstand harsh treatment. Leung et al. (2014) asserted that for individuals recently diagnosed with cancer and undergoing the treatment process, the shock of having cancer, fear of losing their life, feelings of helplessness, and the aggressiveness involved with the treatment of cancer led many to develop signs and experience symptoms of depression that eventuated in posttraumatic stress; however, the patients' confidence after diagnosis and the subsequent resilience in treatment amounts to posttraumatic growth. This would suggest that resilience mediates posttraumatic growth.

In order to gain an increased understanding of the extent to which survivors are able to transcend the trauma associated with diagnosis and treatment of cancer, and develop posttraumatic growth, it is helpful to examine longitudinal studies that examine this association. Costanzo et al. (2009) studied whether cancer survivors demonstrated impairment, resilience, and/or growth. Mental health functioning, mood, psychological wellbeing, social wellbeing, and the impact of aging on psychosocial adjustment were also investigated in 398 cancer survivors, who were participants in the Midlife in the United States (MIDUS) survey, as compared to 796 respondents with no cancer history. Within this longitudinal study, participants who ranged from 24 to 75 years of age responded to an initial telephone survey and self-administered assessments in 1995-96 and again in 2004-06. Symptoms of major depressive disorder, generalized anxiety disorder, and panic disorder were assessed with the World Mental Health Organization Composite International Diagnostic Interview Short Form (WHO CIDI-SF; Kessler et al., 1998) via telephone interview. In measuring positive and negative affect, two 6-item self-administered questionnaires were created based upon several well-validated surveys. Positive psychological functioning was assessed with measures of wellbeing (Ryff & Keyes, 1995) deemed relevant to cancer: environmental mastery, personal growth, positive relations with others, and self-acceptance. Social wellbeing was assessed by meaningfulness of society, social integration, acceptance of others, social contribution, and social actualization (Keyes, 1998). Four scales assessed domains of religiosity and spirituality: the Religious Identification Scale, the Spirituality Scale, the Private Religious Practices Scale, and the Religious Identification and Spirituality Scales.

Results of the Costanzo et al. (2009) study suggested that, following cancer diagnosis and during treatment, cancer survivors demonstrated impairments relative to the comparison group in terms of mental health functioning, mood, and some aspects of psychological wellbeing as compared to an age, gender, and education-matched sample of respondents with no cancer history. Persons who endorsed the most significant decline in mental health functioning during treatment were respondents who reported poorer psychological functioning before diagnosis. For the purpose of this study, resilience was defined as possessing a great degree of social well-being, spirituality, and personal growth pre versus post diagnosis, which suggests resilience was assessed as trait both pre-diagnosis and post-diagnosis. The longitudinal analysis (pre-and post-diagnosis) revealed that cancer survivors rated themselves as experiencing greater resiliency in areas of social wellbeing, spirituality, and personal growth compared to healthy controls. Analysis of pre-diagnosis and post-diagnosis data revealed that persons who endorsed greater levels of psychopathology before cancer diagnosis were more likely to be diagnosed with later cancer. The findings of Costanzo et al. (2009) suggest that cancer survivors endorse resiliency in the long term, although the study did not assess whether adverse experiences before breast cancer contributed to resiliency.

The notion that persons who are able to adapt to unfavorable circumstances which helps in confronting future challenges is not novel. In a longitudinal study, Dooley et al. (2017) analyzed the relationship between lifetime stress exposure before cancer diagnosis and psychological functioning after a breast cancer diagnosis. Because Seery et al., (2010) previously reported that adults who experienced low-to-moderate levels of lifetime stress exposure had better mental health as compared to those with either no or high levels of lifetime stress, they wanted to examine whether toughening effects of moderate stress exposure differed from acute versus chronic stress exposure (Dooley et al., 2017). After potential subjects were excluded due to metastatic disease, the study included 185 women diagnosed with breast cancer. As in indicated in Dooley et al., (2017), the Stress and Adversity Inventory (STRAIN; Bower et al., 2014; Slavich & Toussaint, 2014; Toussaint et al., 2016) was utilized to assess lifetime stress, both acute and chronic. Cancer-related intrusive thoughts were assessed with the Impact of Events Scale (Horowitz et al., 1979). The Positive and Negative Affect Schedule (Watson et al., 1988) assessed both positive and negative affect (Dooley et al., 2017).

They found a significant quadratic relationship between acute stress count and cancer-related intrusions which revealed that participants who experienced a moderate number of acute stressors reported less frequent cancer-related intrusive thoughts, compared with those with a low or high acute stress count (Dooley et al., 2017). Further, there was a significant quadratic relationship between acute stress count and positive affect, indicating that individuals with a moderate number of lifetime acute stressors reported more positive affect, as compared to those with a low or high acute stress count. The operational definition of resilience related to adaptation as the capacity to resume premorbid level of psychological wellbeing. The authors concluded that a moderate lifetime stress exposure was associated with psychological resilience among breast cancer survivors. Specifically, unlike acute stress exposure, chronic stress exposure was not related to intrusive thoughts or positive affect in a quadratic fashion, suggesting that the potential toughening effects of stress exposure may be unique to acute as opposed to chronic stress. The authors posited that moderate stress exposure before breast cancer diagnosis might enable persons to be better prepared to deal with anxiety associated with the breast cancer diagnosis and treatment. One of the limitations of this study is that it did not examine whether past stressors, such as adverse experiences of childhood, impacted the growth experiences of breast cancer survivors.

Taylor et al. (1984) analyzed sense of control and psychological adjustment of women who had undergone breast cancer treatment. Specifically, they hypothesized that breast cancer patients would attribute breast cancer to a specific cause, and that the attributions would be made shortly after breast cancer diagnosis. The reason for this study was to explore whether attributing breast cancer to a specific cause would result in a sense of control as related to health outcomes. Although the study did not indicate the length in time since subject's last treatment, women who experienced chronic medical issues other than breast cancer, and those who had a history of premorbid depression and mental health treatment were excluded from the study. The final sample included 78 women that ranged in age from 29 to 78, with a median age of 53. Participants underwent both a telephone interview with a psychologist, and they also completed rating forms. Factor analysis was completed based upon the following measures: the physician's Global Adjustment to Illness Scale (GAIS) rating; the interviewer's GAIS rating; the respondent's self-rating of current adjustment (5-point scale); the respondent's self-report of current psychological distress (i.e., summed 4-point ratings of degree of anxiety, fear, depression, and anger); the total score of the Profile of Mood States; the Campbell Index of Well-Being score; the significant other's rating of the respondent's adjustment (5-point scale); the Rosenberg Self-Esteem Scale; the Locke-Wallace (1959) Marital Adjustment Scale; and the respondent's self-rating of her coping in comparison with other women (6-point scale). The results indicated that 95% of subjects attributed their breast cancer condition to a specific cause; however, only 23% of participants made this assumption shortly after diagnosis. More relevant to the current study, psychological adjustment was positively associated with a sense of control, $p < .02$. Respondents were also asked if they had made any changes in their lives since the cancer, and 70% reported that cancer had made them think about their lives differently. Positive change was endorsed by 60% of subjects who reported changes. The most commonly reported change concerned learning to take life more easily and to enjoy it more. The authors opined that these changes served as a relative approximation of cognitive control, which were significantly related to adjustment in a positive way, $F(2, 67) = 4.09, p < .03$.

Relationship Between Resilience and Posttraumatic Growth

There is evidence in the literature that although resilience and posttraumatic growth were developed as separate constructs, literature review suggests a relationship between the two. Specifically, persons who are able to meet struggles with a high degree of resilience are able to achieve growth because they are mentally stronger for the experience. Li et al. (2020) analyzed whether resilience was a mediator of anxiety, depression, and posttraumatic growth among breast cancer patients undergoing chemotherapy. The study comprised 260 breast cancer patients who underwent treatment in the breast surgery ward of the First Hospital of Shanxi Medical University in China. The Posttraumatic Growth Inventory (Tedeschi & Calhoun, 1996) was utilized to measure posttraumatic growth's primary outcome variable. Participants completed rating forms in relation to symptoms of anxiety and depression. The Connor-Davidson Resilience Scale (Connor & Davidson, 2003) was translated into Mandarin by Yu and Zhang (2007). The Connor-Davidson Scale was specifically designed as a measure of resilience following traumatic events, indicating that this is a measure of state resilience (Khoshouei, 2009).

The cross-sectional study of Li et al. (2020) was completed from November 2017 to January 2019 and results revealed a significant positive correlation between resilience and posttraumatic growth in breast cancer survivors. Further, in addition to posttraumatic growth, resilience showed a significant negative correlation with anxiety and depression (all p's $< .01$). Resilience had a positively predictive effect on PTG and the standardized estimate of the path coefficient was 0.253 ($P <.05$). Anxiety and depression were negatively predictive of PTG in an indirect manner with resilience as a mediator and the standardized estimate of path coefficient was –0.223 ($P <.05$). The overall effect of anxiety and depression on PTG was –0.321 ($P <.05$), and the direct effect was –0.223 ($P <.05$). The authors opined that the effect of anxiety and depression on PTG could be partially buffered by the mediating of resilience, accounting for 30.53% of the total effect (indirect effect/total effect, –0.098/–0.321). Patients who endorsed a high level of resilience and were able to overcome anxiety and depression achieved greater posttraumatic growth rates than those with moderate or low resilience. Although the analysis offered by Li et al. (2020) provides enlightening data, the study did not explore factors that may fortify resilience and lead to favorable posttraumatic growth. Additionally, because this was cross-sectional, not longitudinal, a clear distinction cannot be made.

There are many factors that contribute to the future capacity to develop resilience and posttraumatic growth from a history of adverse experiences in childhood, specifically physical and emotional abuse. This study investigates resilience and PTG in breast cancer survivors with traumatic childhood experiences. From the preceding discussion on the PTG theory and evidence-based literature studies, the PTG theory is appropriate for this study. The PTG theory is focused on describing how people grow psychologically after experiencing traumatic or stressful situations. While not all people experience posttraumatic growth, those who do reported better quality of life, as evidenced by renewed appreciation for life, new possibilities, personal strength, and increased spirituality. Therefore, in the current study, Tedeschi's Posttraumatic Growth Inventory is used to measure PTG among breast cancer survivors with a traumatic childhood and there is a comparison of the findings to those who have not had such experiences; hence, this study tests the suitability of the PTG theory as a theoretical framework.

Abuse Defined

Child abuse involves the emotional, sexual, physical, or neglect of a child under 18 by a parent, custodian, or caregiver that results in potential harm, harm, or a threat of harm (Shonkoff, 2016). According to the *Child Welfare Survey* put forth by the U.S. Department of Health and Human Services (2022), there were 618,000 victims of child abuse and neglect nationally. It is estimated that for every report of child abuse, two cases of childhood remain unreported (Sharma et al., 2021). Age, gender, and socioeconomic status place children at increased risk for abuse (Shonkoff, 2016).

Physical Abuse

"Physical abuse is generally defined as any nonaccidental physical injury to the child and can include striking, kicking, burning, or biting the child, or any action that results in a physical impairment of the child" (Child Welfare Information Gateway [CWIG], 2019, p. 2). Physical abuse is marked by an intentional physical assault or a person's action that causes or could reasonably be expected to cause physical harm to the child (Norman et al., 2012). Physical abuse also entails excessive force in child discipline. It further involves a failure of preventing a child from harming themself or others. As a nation, the United States of America has no unified definition of abuse. Amongst states, legal definitions of physical abuse vary. For instance, some states do not consider corporal punishment abusive if the child is not harmed, whereas other states consider excessive corporal punishment abusive (CWIG, 2014).

Emotional Abuse

"Injury to the psychological capacity or emotional stability of the child as evidenced by an observable or substantial change in behavior, emotional response, or cognition and injury as evidenced by anxiety, depression, withdrawal, or aggressive behavior" (Child Welfare Information Gateway, 2019, p. 3). Emotional abuse occurs when the actions or omissions, such as scapegoating, rejection, verbal attacks, threats, insults, and humiliation, cause a serious, negative emotional impact on a child (Berger et al., 2015). When emotional abuse is chronic and persistent, it can cause long-term emotional harm to the child.

Association Between Abuse and Breast Cancer

There are decades of empirical work that demonstrate a positive correlation between childhood abuse and negative health consequences. In recent years, studies have shown a positive association between childhood abuse and cancer. In particular, Hovdestad et al. (2020) utilized data from the 2012 Canadian Community Health Survey-Mental Health to examine whether adverse experiences during childhood place persons at risk for developing cancer in adulthood. Retrospective reports of abuse explored associations on three types of childhood maltreatment: physical abuse (CPA), childhood sexual abuse (CSA), and childhood exposure to intimate partner violence (CEIPV). The sample consisted of 9,783 men and 12,132 women ages 18 years and older. The items for CPA and CEIPV were from the Childhood Experiences of Violence Questionnaire (CEVQ). The CSA items were similar to those used in the 2009 Canadian General Social Survey. Results indicated a positive relationship between childhood physical and emotional abuse and cancer for women but not men. When smoking, life stress, depression, and alcohol were included in the models along with age and other sociodemographic variables, childhood physical abuse and childhood emotional abuse continued to be associated with cancer for women, although the relationships were decreased. The most reported form of abuse among cancer patients was childhood physical abuse (21.4% of women and 31.1% of men). Further, with greater frequency and severity of childhood physical abuse, there was an increase in cancer diagnoses, specifically in women (2.5%). Childhood sexual abuse was reported by 14.4% of women and 5.9% of men, and childhood emotional abuse was reported by 9.0% of women and 6.7% of men. Sociodemographic characteristics and cancer risk factors mediated the association between women's retrospective reports of CSA and cancer. Although this study highlights an association between childhood maltreatment and potential development of cancer, it did not examine the relationship of childhood adverse experiences with resilience and posttraumatic growth in breast cancer survivors.

Apart from problematic alcohol consumption as a mediating variable between childhood abuse and increased cancer risk, previous research has identified chronic inflammation as another risk factor. Generally, inflammation is a physiological response of the body against injuries, toxins, and infections (Ports et al., 2019). However, prolonged chronic inflammation may trigger genetic mutation, resulting in the development of malignant tumors at the inflammation sites (Chen & Lacey, 2018). In the existing literature, researchers have hypothesized that persons with a history of adverse childhood experiences are prone to chronic stress disorders in their adult lives (Chen & Lacey, 2018). Stress, in turn, activates the sympathetic nervous system, which triggers inflammation, subsequently increasing their risk of developing cancers. While some persons with a history of childhood maltreatment develop chronic stress-related disorders, others learn to adapt to adverse experiences of childhood with resilience. The capacity to determine resiliency in response to abusive experiences during childhood has been associated with greater levels of resilience later in life (Fritz et al., 2018).

Fritz et al. (2018) completed a metanalytic study of social, emotional, cognitive, and/or behavioral resilience factors after childhood adversity. The analysis consisted of longitudinal studies in which the resilience was assessed before psychopathology, and childhood adverse experiences was measured no later than the resiliency factors. For the purpose of this study, psychopathology was defined as general mental distress, as self-harm behavior, as suicidal ideation, or as categorical diagnosis or continuous symptoms of any disorder included within the DSM-IV-TR, and over 200 studies met criteria. A total of 15 childhood adverse experiences were identified. Therefore, the authors determined a second set of criteria wherein the resilience factor was required to function as moderator and/or mediator for the relationship between childhood adverse experiences and psychopathology, which consisted of 22 studies Based upon the heterogenous nature of the 22 studies, a quantitative analysis was deemed inappropriate, and therefore, a qualitative analysis was completed. The review revealed that 13 of the 22 articles determined individual factors that were associated with resilience including three cognitive, four emotion regulation, three social interaction/attachment, and three personality/self-concept RFs. The cognitive factors most highly associated with resilience were stronger intellect and cognitive restructuring. In terms of emotional regulation, high distress tolerance, low expressive suppression, low aggression, and low alcohol coping expectancy were associated with resilience. Low insecure attachment, low disconnection/rejection, and low other-directedness were positively associated with resilience. In the personality/self-concept domain, a balance between low and high ego control, and high self-esteem was positively associated with resilience.

Although there is an association between childhood adverse experiences and breast cancer, there are more common causes of breast cancer than childhood abuse. After the primary risk factor of gender, the substantial risk factor is age, in that each year beyond the age of 50, women are more likely to develop breast cancer (Momenimovahed & Salehiniya, 2019). Another significant risk factor is blood type, specifically women with blood group A and Rhesus positive have a higher risk of developing breast cancer, while women with blood group AB and Rhesus negative have a lower risk of developing breast cancer. There are several reproductive factors that correlate with developing breast cancer such as younger age of menarche onset, onset of menopause after the age of 50, having more than five full-term pregnancies, and advanced maternal age at the time of the first pregnancy. There are also several hormonal factors that place women at risk for developing breast cancer such as birth control pills, ovulation-stimulating drugs, and postmenopausal hormone therapy, which are all associated with increased risk for breast cancer. Lastly, yet significant, approximately 40% of hereditary breast cancer cases occur due to mutations in the BRCA1 and BRCA2 genes (Momenimovahed & Salehiniya, 2019).

Overall, although there is an association between adverse experiences in childhood and breast cancer, there are numerous biological factors that place women at greater risk for breast cancer as opposed to abuse. Because of the complexity of the impact of childhood adverse experiences (AEs), a specific odds ratio for women with a history of childhood AEs (as opposed to biological factors) has yet to be determined. Barber et al. (2021) did find that Black women with a history of chronic lifetime stress were 25% more likely to be diagnosed with hormone receptor positive breast cancer. Nonetheless, because women with a history of childhood abuse possess some increased likelihood of developing breast cancer, it is important to determine whether the same adverse experiences in childhood either contribute to or inhibit their ability to meet the challenges of breast cancer with resilience, and ultimately develop posttraumatic growth.

Posttraumatic Growth and Childhood Abuse

Traumatic events can be severe to the extent that there may be minimal or no posttraumatic growth. In some instances, persons with a history of childhood abuse may develop some posttraumatic growth even when the impact of trauma has not fully resolved. Mohr and Rosén (2017) studied whether protective factors moderated the relationship between childhood adverse experiences and later posttraumatic growth. Participants included 501 university students, 250 of whom endorsed a history of some form of adverse experience during childhood. Developed for this study was the Maltreatment History Survey (MHS), which assesses physical abuse, sexual abuse, emotional abuse, and neglect. The Posttraumatic Growth Inventory (PTGI; Tedeschi & Calhoun, 1996) measured posttraumatic growth. The PTGI contains 21 items relating to positive outcomes following trauma. As cited within Mohr and Rosén (2017), the Social and Emotional Resources Inventory (SERI; Mohr & Rosén, 2012) was utilized to assess protective factors and the degree to which these are present. The SERI contains 50 items that measure individual, familial, and community protective factors. It comprises 12 subscales, including intelligence, parenting practices, parent connections, self-esteem, money, resources, faith, talent, good schools, prosocial adults, kin connections, and prosocial organizations.

Mohr and Rosén (2017) reported that, of participants with a history of childhood abuse and neglect, 236 (91%) endorsed some level of posttraumatic growth. The most common themes that emerged were perceived growth related to improving relationships, enhanced empathy, exploring new areas of interest, a sense of independence, a commanding sense of power and control, and feeling grateful for life. Data analysis revealed that the only variables that significantly predicted posttraumatic growth were acceptance, emotional support, and positive reframing. This study focused on posttraumatic growth following adverse experiences during childhood, but did not assess resiliency and posttraumatic growth when confronted with other adverse experiences during adulthood, such as breast cancer.

This study suggests that some forms of adverse childhood experiences may promote the development of a sense of autonomy, and a sense of strength, and agency. These traits may then assist in the management of subsequent challenges, such as with the trauma of breast cancer diagnosis and treatment.

Impact of Abuse Severity

In addition to the type of abuse, abuse severity may also affect whether these early adverse experiences promote resilience and growth or increase psychopathology. The literature reviewed reflects that a history of some adversity challenges persons to utilize their resilience in order to adapt. Consistent with Dooley et al. (2017), however, persons with a history of more severe abuse are more likely to feel overwhelmed emotionally. The development of severe psychopathology that is associated with severe abuse may leave individuals unable to utilize and develop further resilience. Those with limited resilience are then not likely to be able to engage in posttraumatic growth when faced with later potentially traumatic challenges, such as breast cancer.

Summary

Some women endorse a sense of personal growth following their experience of breast cancer treatment. Other survivors either do not feel emotionally stronger, or they persist with the anxiety they experienced during treatment. There appear to be many factors that may contribute to a breast cancer survivor's experiencing resilience and posttraumatic growth. A common theme for women who achieve resilience and posttraumatic growth in the long term is that they suffer from anxiety during treatment, but then they are able to successfully transcend the emotional difficulties. Further, prior studies have established that persons who adapt to unfavorable circumstances are more amenable to developing growth when confronting future challenges. One such challenge is childhood abuse. While there is an abundance of research that outlines that negative mental health outcomes of childhood physical and emotional abuse, there is a gap in the literature as to whether resilience and growth experienced from childhood trauma aids in developing positive long-term adjustment to the emotional trauma of breast cancer. This study aims to examine the relationship of resilience and posttraumatic growth and adverse childhood abuse experiences in breast cancer survivors. Posttraumatic growth theory developed by Tedeschi and Calhoun (1995) is the framework for the current study. To understand whether some types of early life abusive experience yield resilience and posttraumatic growth, this investigation utilizes measures of retrospective report of abuse, resiliency, and posttraumatic growth.

CHAPTER THREE: STATEMENT OF THE PROBLEM

The problem of focus in this study is the unknown impact of physical and emotional abuse in childhood on the adult lives of breast cancer survivors. Evidence from existing literature indicates several negative outcomes associated with adverse childhood experiences (Mandelli et al., 2015). Some of the negative effects that manifest in the adult lives of individuals include the development of stress and depression, as well as a greater likelihood of developing lifestyle diseases (Dooley et al., 2017).

While there is substantial theoretical information that details the lifelong ill psychological effects of childhood maltreatment, a literature review reveals this history of maltreatment may also strengthen resiliency and yield some level of posttraumatic growth. Therefore, it is worth questioning whether the resiliency and posttraumatic growth harnessed through adverse childhood experiences will promote some level of resiliency and posttraumatic growth with breast cancer survival. Breast cancer can alone be deemed traumatic, so it is reasonable to discern whether experience working through previous trauma leads to skill in healing from subsequent trauma (Brandão et al., 2017). Such questions are relevant because the resultant data may be useful in determining whether breast cancer survivors would benefit from psychological care to enhance resiliency and promote posttraumatic growth. Further, this study may lead to a greater understanding of how childhood experiences may be harnessed in order to optimize resiliency and posttraumatic growth. Because the severity of adverse experiences during childhood can either thwart or contribute to the associated level of resiliency and posttraumatic growth, it is important to consider the severity of abuse when examining these issues.

While most past scholars have mainly focused on the negative effects of adverse experiences, a few have attempted to examine resiliency among breast cancer survivors.

Literature review reveals there is an association between developing resilience and posttraumatic growth following breast cancer treatment (Guil et al., 2020). There is also evidence that resilience is a mediator between depression/anxiety and posttraumatic growth. The current study fills a gap in the literature about a lack of research and knowledge on how adverse childhood experiences affect breast cancer survivors' resiliency and posttraumatic growth.

Purpose of the Study

It is important to understand whether milder abusive experiences lead to greater resilience, because this resilience can be utilized therapeutically. Strengthening resilience is an important therapeutic tool (Schulz et al., 2014). This study aims to examine the impact of early physical and emotional abuse during childhood on resilience and posttraumatic growth following breast cancer survival. The independent variables of interest in the study are perceived childhood physical abuse and perceived emotional abuse. The dependent variables are resiliency and posttraumatic growth among breast cancer survivors. The target population in the study includes female breast cancer survivors. Part of the stratified sample includes female breast cancer survivors who have a prior history of childhood adversity. The rest of the sample includes female breast cancer survivors who do not have a history of childhood adversity. A quantitative sample has been extracted from this target population for this study. The geographical delimitation of the study is in the United States.

The conceptual model is that resilience partially mediates the effects of abuse severity on PTG in women who have been diagnosed with breast cancer 2 or more years prior to the present time. Figure 1 depicts the hypothesized associations between the core variables under consideration in the current investigation. As seen in Figure 1, the model proposes that resilience mediates the association between physical/emotional abuse severity and PTG among breast cancer survivors.

Figure 1

The Hypothesized Relationship of Resilience as a Mediator Between Physical/Emotional Abuse Severity and Posttraumatic Growth

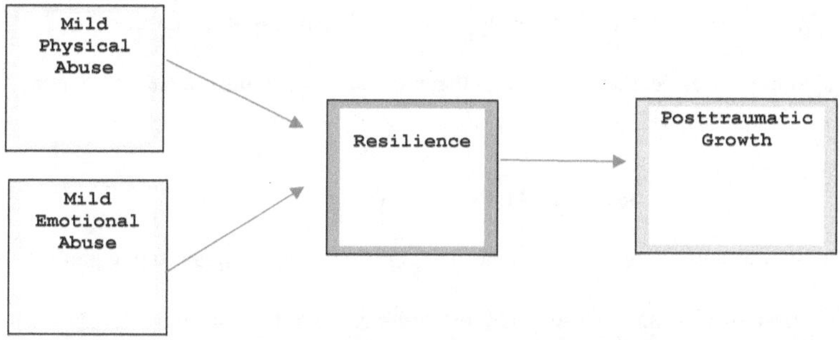

Research Questions and Hypotheses

RQ1: Does perceived abuse during childhood have a significant impact on measures of resiliency and posttraumatic growth among breast cancer survivors?

H1: Mild physical/emotional abuse during childhood will be associated with greater levels of posttraumatic growth than either no abuse or more severe levels of abuse.

H2: Mild physical/emotional abuse will be associated with greater levels of resilience than either no abuse or more severe levels of abuse.

H3: Resilience will be positively associated with posttraumatic growth. In other words, breast cancer survivors with higher levels of resilience will report higher levels of posttraumatic growth.

H4: Resilience will mediate the association between emotional abuse and posttraumatic growth.

CHAPTER FOUR: METHODOLOGY

Introduction

The chapter begins with a review of the research method and design adopted, then a discussion of participants' selection procedures. The chapter also includes a review of the instruments that were used for collecting and data. In the fourth section, I present details on the data collection procedures that were used. Lastly, there is a discussion of the data analysis procedures used alongside ethical considerations that were adhered to during collection and analysis of the data.

Research Method and Design

A quantitative research method was used in the current study. A quantitative method emphasizes operationalization and measurement of variables such that data generated are in a numerical format (Lazaraton, 2005). A quantitative method also involves analyzing numerical data through computational or statistical techniques. The end goal of this analysis was to statistically describe variables of interest or measure causal and non-causal associations among variables (Lazaraton, 2005),

A quantitative method was suitable because the purpose of the current study was to examine a relationship between childhood abuse and resiliency/posttraumatic growth. The research purpose and objective can be decomposed into specific measurable variables, childhood abuse and resiliency/PTG. Since the variables of interest can be operationalized and measured, associations among them can be established using appropriate statistical techniques. There are limitations with cross-sectional designs, such as used in the present study as compared to longitudinal designs. Longitudinal studies are more reliable in addressing both systematic method error due to the use of a single rater or single source, as well as causal inference

(Rindfleisch et al, 2008). Because a longitudinal study was not possible, a cross-sectional design was appropriate because the study was theoretical and several measurement instruments were utilized.

Participants

Target Population

The target population for the current study included female breast cancer survivors in the United States. According to the American Cancer Society (2022), there were over 3.8 million female breast cancer survivors in the United States by April 2022. This number included women that had completed treatment and those that were still participating in treatment but on their path to recovery. The American Cancer Society (2022) further estimated that about one in 39 women dies from breast cancer in the United States, translating into a mortality rate of 2.6%. In another observation, Stump-Sutliff (2022) indicated that the 5-year survival rate for women with breast cancer is 90%, while the 10-year survival rate is 84% (Stump-Sutliff, 2022). The 15-year survival rate is slightly lower, although still an impressive figure when compared to other cancers (80%; Stump-Sutliff, 2022). The large number of breast cancer survivors in the United States provides a large pool from which participants can be selected for inclusion in this study.

After securing IRB approval, a Qualtrics survey was administered to breast cancer survivors who received a breast cancer diagnosis more than 2 years, and up to 25 years prior to the present time. I have joined several breast cancer forums on social media platforms, and I am an active member of both the Pennsylvania Breast Cancer Coalition and the Susan B. Komen Foundation, where I offered the survey. The current study is comprised of adult females over the age of 18 years.

Inclusion and Exclusion Criteria

The following inclusion and exclusion criteria were used to identify and select eligible participants for this study:

- Participants were of legal consenting age of at least 18 years of age.
- Because this study examined resiliency and posttraumatic growth in breast cancer survivors, all participants were breast cancer survivors (history of a breast cancer diagnosis).
- Participants were assigned female at birth.
- Participants were at least 2 years out from the initial breast cancer diagnosis. This is because this study examined resiliency and posttraumatic growth in the long term.
- The study includes survivors of all breast cancer stages, and therefore some survivors may still be receiving treatment when completing the survey.
- Survivors may have had other cancers, and/or breast cancer recurrence.

Measurement/Instruments

Background Information Questionnaire

Demographic Information and Breast Cancer History

The Background Information Questionnaire (Appendix D) was the instrument used to gather a wide variety of information that was useful to this study. Further, it served to delineate results that were pertinent to this study, while also examining aspects of the data that were not being focused on in this study. Thus, these data may be used for future studies. Demographic data included age, educational attainment, current employment/number of jobs, income, marital status/number of marriages, religion, spirituality, and number of persons in household. Additionally, respondents were questioned with respect to history of mental health treatment.

Respondents were also questioned with respect to length of time since breast cancer diagnosis, as well as breast cancer staging.

Health-Related Quality of Life

The Research and Development (RAND) 36-Item Health Survey 1.0 Questionnaire was used as a health-related quality of life measure (Ware & Sherbourne, 1992). RAND grants public use of the survey in accordance with specific terms and conditions. The 35-item, standardized health-related quality of life measures helped control for health-related factors, both relating to long-term effects of breast cancer, as well as other non-breast cancer-related health issues. Items are based upon eight health concepts: physical functioning, bodily pain, role limitations due to physical health problems, role limitations due to personal or emotional problems, emotional well-being, social functioning, energy/fatigue, and general health perceptions. The RAND Health Survey also includes one item relating to perceived change in health. As indicated in Ware & Sherbourne (1992), test items were adapted from longer instruments completed by patients participating in the Medical Outcomes Study (MOS; Hays & Shapiro, 1992; Stewart, Sherbourne, Hays, et al., 1992), an observational study of variations in physician practice styles and patient outcomes in different systems of health care delivery (Hays & Shapiro, 1993). The original MOS study included both a cross-sectional and a longitudinal element. For the cross-sectional component, over 20,000 patients were sampled from among adults visiting participating practices during 9-day health screening periods in 1986. Patients from the cross-sectional study had one or more of four chronic medical conditions: hypertension, diabetes, heart disease, or depression. Participants from the cross-sectional study constituted the sampling frame for the longitudinal panel of 2,546 patients (Ware & Sherbourne, 1992).

Items range from binary, yes-no, to 4-item, 5-item, and 6-item, Likert scales. A total score on the RAND 36-Item Health Survey 1.0 Questionnaire ranges from 0 to 100, with a higher score reflecting more favorable health (Ware & Sherbourne, 1992). Scores represent the percentage of total possible score achieved. Additionally, items within respective scales are averaged to create the 8 scaled scores. Omitted items that are left blank are not taken into account when calculating the scale scores. Therefore, scale scores represent the average for all items completed. The RAND pain scale score correlated 0.99 in the MOS panel sample at baseline with a mean difference of 3.33 (SF-36 lower on average), standard deviation of 3.38, and range of differences from - 8 to +10 ($n = 2224$). These results suggest that although scoring differences for an individual patient can be fairly large (0.39 of a standard deviation), the effects on central tendency estimates and rank order for the MOS longitudinal panel tend to be minimal. In regard to the general health scale, scores correlated 0.99 in the MOS panel sample at baseline with a standard error of measurement of -1. 37, standard deviation of 0.98 \(Ware & Sherbourne, 1992).). Data were from baseline of the Medical Outcomes Study ($N = 2471$). According to Burnam et al. (1988), "depressed" is defined by the 8-item depression symptom scale. The following scales did not differ significantly (.05) from one another: 1- physical functioning, females, not depressed, and males not depressed; 2- role functioning/physical, females not depressed, and males depressed and not depressed; 3- role functioning/emotional, males not depressed; 4- emotional/fatigue, females not depressed and depressed, and males not depressed and depressed; 5- emotional wellbeing, males not depressed; 6- social functioning, females not depressed and depressed, and males not depressed and depressed; 7- pain, females not depressed and depressed, and males not depressed and depressed; and, 8- general health, females not depressed and depressed, and males not depressed and depressed (Ware & Sherbourne, 1992).

Breast Cancer Quality of Life Measure

Respondents were questioned with respect to breast cancer-related worry, fatigue, impact on work, matters of wellbeing, which can impact data outcomes. The BREAST-Q 2.0 core scales were used as a breast cancer treatment outcome measure (Klassen et al., 2021). The BREAST-Q is a copyrighted survey which, according to the licensing agreement, can be used free of charge for non-profit purposes including research. The BREAST-Q 2.0 is a patient-reported outcome measure (PROM) designed to evaluate outcomes among women undergoing different types of breast surgery. BREAST-Q was initially published in 2009 (Pusic et al., 2009) and then revised, 2.0 version (Klassen et al., 2021). The original BREAST-Q was only comprised of two scales, Psychological Wellbeing and Sexual Wellbeing. In creating the revised scale, qualitative interviews were completed with 57 breast cancer patients pre and post-surgery, adjuvant, and neoadjuvant treatment. The additional scales of cancer worry, fatigue, and impact on work were then established and field tested in Love Research Army (LRA) sample (n= 1,680), 1,006 of whom completed a test-retest. Reliability was > 0.81 for the person separation index, > 0.89 for Cronbach's alpha, and > 0.83 for interclass correlation coefficients. Lower scores on all three scales were significantly associated with being closer in time to diagnosis and having a higher cancer stage at diagnosis ($p < 0.001$ on ANOVA; Klassen et al., 2021).

The BREAST-Q 2.0 is a 44-item scale comprised of the following composite scores: psychological wellbeing, sexual wellbeing, cancer worry, fatigue, and impact on work (Klassen et al., 2021). Psychological wellbeing items assess level of confidence, acceptance, and sense of normalcy. Sexual wellbeing measures feelings of attractiveness clothed and unclothed, sexual confidence, and satisfaction. Cancer worry assesses anxiety with respect to fear of death, cancer spreading, bodily damage due to treatment, impact on activities of daily living, and similar fears.

The fatigue scale assesses mobility limitations, and the impact of fatigue as related to completing chores, maintaining alertness, participating in social activities, and mood stability. Impact on work addresses work limitations regarding the need for assistance, diminished work performance, and reduction of hours and/or responsibilities (Klassen et al., 2021).

Responses are completed on a 1-4, Likert Scale on the work, worry, and fatigue scales. Responses range from 1, *strongly disagree* to 4, *strongly agree* (Klassen et al., 2021). Responses are endorsed on a 1-5 Likert Scale on the psychological wellbeing and on the sexual wellbeing scales. Responses range from 1, *none of the time*, to 5, *all of the time*. BREAST-Q does not yield a total composite score; rather scores are tabulated for each of the 5 scales. To score a scale, the raw scores for the set of respective items are added, which produces a total raw score. When less than 50% of a scale's data is missing, a mean of the completed items is calculated prior to computing the total raw score. The total raw score for the scale is then converted to a score that ranges from 0 to 100. Higher scores for all BREAST-Q scales, with the exception of the cancer worry scale, reflect a better outcome (Klassen et al., 2021).

Abuse Measure

The Emotional and Physical Abuse Questionnaire (EPAB; Carlin et al., 1994) is a non-copyrighted retrospective measure of specific experiences of discipline and abuse during childhood. Using a 6-point Likert scale (0 = *Never to* 5 = *Very Frequently*), respondents indicate frequency for each item that translates into indications of abuse on a scale from mild to severe. The EPAB has 37 items that pertain to researcher definitions of abuse with 2 additional items asking respondents whether they self-define themselves as having been physically or emotionally abused. These two questions were moved to the background information questionnaire in order to avoid an issue of bias (Wolkins, 2020). For the purpose of this study, analysis was based upon the 14 physical abuse items, in addition to the four emotional abuse items. The remaining (19 items) pertain to neglect and discipline, which are not being assessed in this study.

The EPAB is a widely used measure of abuse and has been used by Doherty et al. (2022), Wolkins (2020), Asaro et al. (2019), Nagy et al. (2019), and Quintana (2014). The EPAB has strong parametric properties, possibly the reason for its widespread use. Coefficient alpha reliability rates for physical abuse assessment are .81 for non-Asian men and .82 for non-Asian women, .76 for Asian men, and .80 for Asian women (Meston et al., 1999). The EPAB provides measurement of (a) researcher definition of childhood physical abuse, (b) researcher definition of childhood emotional abuse, (c) subjective definition of childhood physical abuse, and (d) subjective definition of childhood emotional abuse.

The current study highlighted both subjective, self-defined abuse and researcher-defined abuse, because there is some evidence that abuse perception does not solely impact adjustment (Linde-Krieger et al., 2021). Silvern et al. (2000) found that researcher-defined abuse is associated with more severe outcomes than survivor-defined abuse (Linde-Krieger et al, 2021). Findings of several studies suggest that researcher definition of childhood physical abuse is a predictor of adult psychopathology after controlling for subjective definition of childhood physical abuse (Carlin et al., 1994; Goldsmith et al., 2009; Knutson & Selner, 1994; Rausch & Knutson, 1991; Silvern et al., 2000). A limitation with this research is the inability to obtain an adequate sample of participants who meet criteria for subjective definition of childhood physical abuse. Thus, the most inclusive means of analyzing childhood abuse is to rely upon both research defined and subjective recall of abuse.

Researcher-Defined Abuse Measure

The purpose of using a researcher-defined abuse measure is because persons may not perceive a history of abusive experiences, when in fact the conditions they endured qualify as abuse based upon researcher definitions. One of the advantages of the EPAB is that it allows a researcher to objectively determine if a respondent has experienced physical or emotional abuse by asking about discipline. Although respondents may not perceive abuse, based upon parameters for specific questions at a determined point on the Likert scale, this serves as means of determining whether abuse occurred (by way of discipline) even when respondents answer "no" to abuse questions. There were two forms of abuse measured: physical and emotional abuse.

Researcher-Defined Physical Abuse

Using a researcher definition of childhood physical abuse is often preferable as it is an objective measure that allows for a standardized and quantifiable outcome that can be reliably compared across responders and studies (Velentgas et al., 2013). Studies based upon researcher-defined childhood physical abuse have provided understanding of cause and effect, intervention methods, and mechanisms for both controlling and preventing abuse. Many theoretical explanations and etiological models have been developed. However, contradictions in the findings have also surfaced, partly due to the differences in operationalization of childhood physical abuse (Muela et al., 2012).

The researcher-defined definition of physical abuse during childhood followed the example set by Carlin et al. (1994). Respondents' answers were coded into an ordinal variable of (0) *not abused,* (1) *mild abuse,* and (2) *abused,* providing a measure of abuse severity. The researcher definition of frequency of childhood physical abuse variable was calculated by averaging the responses of the 14 items, which offered a continuous physical abuse severity index. Carlin et al. (1994) developed the Physical Abuse subscale (PAB) summing the frequency responses to 14 items.

Based on Wolkins (2020) and Carlin et al. (1994), the researcher definition of childhood physical abuse variable was coded into an ordinal variable of either (0) not abused, (1) mildly abused, or (2) abused. This provides a measure of abuse severity. Participants were coded as "mild abuse" if they endorse any frequency of the following three items: "I was spanked or hit," "I was pinched as punishment," or "I was hit or spanked with a belt." Because the incidence of the preceding forms of abuse may have been more culturally acceptable in certain populations than others, the type of abuse is classified as mild. Participants were coded as having been "abused" if they rate any of nine major assault questions on the EPAB with a frequency of 1 or greater ("I have received black eyes from being hit," "I was injured seriously enough by a parent or guardian to require medical care," "I had broken bones following a beating," "I was purposely burned with a cigarette, lighter, iron, etc.," "I was bitten so hard marks were left or my skin was broken," "My hair was snatched or pulled out," "I had teeth loosened or knocked out," "I was strangled or choked," "I was thrown against objects, walls, or downstairs"). Participants were also coded as abused if they rated five items that are not major assault items with a frequency of 3 or greater ("I was pinched as punishment," "I was hit or spanked with a board, stick, or wire," "I was tied up as punishment," "I was hit or spanked with a belt," "I was shaken"). Although these harsher forms of abuse may be more common in certain demographics than others, these types of punishment are still classified as abuse based upon researcher definitions of abuse. All other participants were coded as "not abused". The Physical Abuse subscale (PAB), based on the work of Carlin and colleagues (1994) was used as a measure of researcher definition of frequency of childhood physical abuse. It consists of 14 items that are rated on a 6- point Likert-type scale (0 = *never* to 5 = *very frequently*). These items are (a) "I have received black eyes from being hit," (b) "I was injured seriously enough by a parent or guardian to require medical care," (c) "I have had broken bones following a beating," (d) "I was purposefully burned with a cigarette, lighter, iron, etc.," (e) "I was pinched," (f) "I was bitten so hard marks were left or my skin was broken," (g) "I was hit or spanked with a board, stick, or wire," (h) "I was tied up as punishment," (i) "My hair was snatched or pulled out," (j) "I have had teeth loosened or knocked out," (k) "I was hit or spanked with a belt," (l) "I was strangled or choked," (m) "I was shaken," (n) "I was thrown against objects, walls, or downstairs." The researcher definition 65 of frequency of childhood physical abuse variable were calculated by averaging the responses of the 14 items. This averaged response served as the direct measure of the range of physical abuse severity.

Researcher-Defined Emotional Abuse

The Emotional Abuse subscale (EAB) from the EPAB (Carlin et al., 1994) was used as a measure of researcher-defined frequency of childhood emotional abuse. It consists of 4 items that are rated on a 6-point Likert-type scale (0 = *never* to 5 = *very frequently*). Items include (a) "I was mocked or taunted," (b) "I was ridiculed in front of friends or strangers," (c) "At home I was criticized and made to feel worthless," and (d) "I saw other family members humiliated." The researcher definition of frequency of childhood emotional abuse variable was calculated by averaging the responses of the four items. For the purpose of this analysis, "frequency" translates to "severity." This served as a continuous index of severity based upon the average of the 4 items pertaining to emotional abuse.

The Emotional Abuse subscale (EAB) from the EPAB (Carlin et al., 1994) was used as a measure of researcher-defined frequency of childhood emotional abuse. It consists of four items that are rated on a 6-point Likert-type scale (0 = *never* to 5 = *very frequently*). Items include (a) "I was mocked or taunted," (b) "I was ridiculed in front of friends or strangers," (c) "At home I was criticized and made to feel worthless," and (d) "I saw other family members humiliated." The researcher definition of range of childhood emotional abuse variable was calculated by averaging the responses of the four items.

Self-Defined Abuse Measure

The self-defined abuse measure is contained within the items on the background information questionnaire. For both types of abuse assessed within the survey, there are three explicit, forced-choice questions wherein participants indicate "yes" they were abused or "no" if they were not. The three questions for both types of abuse pertain to whether the abuse occurred (or not) in childhood, adolescence, and/or adulthood. The self-defined measure of abuse is based upon subjective recall. Participants responded to questions with respect to their retrospective recall of abusive experiences. Reuben et al. (2016) completed a longitudinal study on the impact of adverse childhood experiences (ACE) as related to health outcomes in adulthood. Based upon retrospective account, subjects rated the type of abuse they experienced during childhood. Generally, with the increased incidence of more than one type of abuse, adult respondents were more inclined to endorse suboptimal physical health (somatic concerns). Retrospective versus prospective means of assessing the impact of childhood abuse were determined to be more strongly predictive of adult outcomes when outcomes were assessed subjectively. Susser and Widom (2012) determined that retrospective recall of childhood abuse reported during adulthood was highly associated with psychopathology. Mental health dysfunction was more contingent upon subjective report during adulthood versus official records of abuse that are medical, legal, and/or psychological in nature.

Physical Abuse

There are three questions asking for a subjective appraisal of whether they have experienced physical abuse at any time in their life. Those questions are, "I consider myself to have been physically abused as a child (ages 0 to 11)"; "I consider myself to have been physically abused as an adolescent (ages 12 to 17)"; and "I consider myself to have been physically abused as an adult (ages 18 or older)." The questions are binary in nature, meaning the respondent can only endorse yes or no for each question.

Emotional Abuse

The items on the background information inquiring about emotional abuse are structured the same as physical abuse. There are three questions asking for a subjective appraisal of whether they have experienced emotional abuse at any time in their life. Those questions are, "I consider myself to have been emotionally abused as a child (ages 0 to 11)"; "I consider myself to have been emotionally abused as an adolescent (ages 12 to 17)"; and "I consider myself to have been emotionally abused as an adult (ages 18 or older)."

Adult Psychopathology

Although adult psychopathology was not examined within this study, data regarding adult psychopathology were collected, and may be used in future studies. The Symptom Checklist-90 items (SCL-90; non-copyrighted version) evaluated adult psychopathology. The non-copyrighted version SCL-90 is a 90-item self-report symptom inventory designed to measure psychopathology on a 5-point Likert scale, indicating the rate of symptom occurrence (0=*not at all*, 4=*extremely*) (Derogatis, 2000). It measures symptom severity on nine symptom scales:

somatization (SOM), obsessive-compulsive (O-C), interpersonal sensitivity (I-S), depression (DEP), anxiety (ANX), hostility (HOS), phobic anxiety (PHOB), paranoid ideation (PAR), and psychoticism (PSY). The SCL-90 also provides three global indices: Global Severity Index (GSI), Positive Symptom Distress Index (PSDI), and a Positive Symptom Total (PST; Derogatis & Savitz, 1999). The GSI is the mean of all 90 items, the PSDI is the average score of the items scored above zero, and the PST is the number of items scored above zero (Derogatis, 2000). The SCL-90 takes approximately 12 to 20 minutes to complete. The SCL-90 has been empirically supported as a measure of symptom change and symptom change in clinical and nonclinical populations (Derogatis, 2000). The SCL-90 can identify those with and without a psychological disorder and can also reveal gender differences in subjective psychopathology among inpatients (Rytilä-Manninen et al., 2016). The GSI provides the best indicator of the level of presenting psychopathology (Derogatis, 2000). The GSI, not the 9 scales nor the 3 indices, were used as a measure of adult psychopathology.

The SCL-90 reliability measures include internal consistency and test-retest reliability. Internal consistency coefficients (Cronbach's alpha) have been reported across various populations as control groups (Derogatis, 1983), primary care (Derogatis, 2000), stroke patients (Aben et al., 2002), and psychiatric inpatients (Hafkenscheid, 1993). Internal consistency coefficients (Cronbach's alpha) have been reported across control groups (Derogatis, 1983), substance abuse inpatients (Zack, Toneatto, & Streiner, 1998), cancer patients (Fitch et al., 1995), and psychiatric inpatients (Rauter, Leonard, & Swett, 1995). The SCL-90 has acceptable levels of factorial invariance for the dimensions, including gender, high validity for depression, and concurrent validation with the MMPI (Derogatis et al., 1976; Derogatis & Savitz, 1999).

Outcome Measures

The following measures were used to determine levels of resiliency and posttraumatic growth as discussed in this document.

Resilience Measure

The Predictive 6-Factor Resilience Scale (PR6) incorporates domains measured by other resilience scales across six distinct neurobiological constructs associated with resiliency, and it also incorporates a sixth domain of health (Rossouw & Rossouw, 2016). Written permission was granted by the authors provided that these results are shared upon study completion. The PR6 model, a measure of trait resilience, is consistent with other resiliency measures in that adaptation is positively associated with resilience, and neuroplasticity facilitates this adaptation. The PR6 domains, plus additional health factor are as follows (Rossouw & Rossouw, 2016):

1. **Vision**: The ability to engage in self-efficacy and goal setting associated with hopefulness, planning, and positive outlook. The form of resilience relates to state/outcome. The neurobiological underpinnings to the interaction between memory storage and retrieval of the hippocampus and categorizing information based upon meaning by the prefrontal cortex (PFC) plays a part in maintaining a hopeful sense of the future, and this is reinforced by goal directedness (Preston & Eichenbaum, 2013).
2. **Composure:** One's capacity for emotional regulation, self-control, and self-awareness. The neurobiological factors of composure relate to the ability of the insula to effectively interpret signals and enable regulation of the hypothalamic–pituitary–adrenal (HPA) axis (Davidson & Begley, 2012).
3. **Tenacity:** A person's ability to harness and exert perseverance and hardiness in order to overcome adverse circumstances. Most measures consider tenacity the most important

aspect of resilience. From a neurophysiological standpoint, tenacity is associated with the PFC's ability to effectively regulate limbic and HPA activation (Davidson & Begley, 2012).

4. **Reasoning**: This domain is associated with higher-level aspects of resiliency, such as problem-solving, ingenuity, growing through adversity, and continuing to thrive/flourish. The capacity to reason is associated with resilience because problem solving is crucial to learning to adapt. The limbic system regulates motivation, emotion, and learning that support strategies for interpretation bias. The interpretation bias serves as a protective factor that yields a plausible sense of optimism (Clarke et al., 2014; Oettingen & Wadden, 1991).
5. **Collaboration:** Relates to psychosocial interaction, including secure attachment, support networks, context, and humor. Schore (2000) noted that the right prefrontal cortex (RPFC), which receives cues interpreted by other regions, plays a key role in secure attachment.
6. **Momentum:** Measures approach versus avoidance as related to sense of direction and openness to new challenges.
7. **Health:** A measure of overall health hygiene and the ability to engage in self-care.

Reponses to the 16-items report form are endorsed on a 5-point Likert scale ranging from 1 = *not at all like me* (most negative), 2 = *a bit like me*, 3 = *somewhat like me*, 4 = *often like me*, and 5 = *very much like me* (most positive). The PR6 scales for each domain were validated with good internal consistency (>0.70). The PR6-50 showed very high internal consistency (0.9372), while the revised 16-item PR6 showed high internal consistency (0.8398). Resilience results showed a correlation of 0.536 (P value < 0.001) with tenacity, while the Vision domain showed the highest correlation at 0.607 (P value < 0.001).

The psychometric properties of the 16-item short version are similar to the 50-question long version, revealing strong convergent validity (Rossouw et al., 2017). Each domain was averaged to produce a comparable score per domain. An Overall Resilience Score (PR6 score) was calculated as an average of each of the six domains, ranging from 0 (lowest resilience) to 1 (highest resilience). The distribution of PR6 scores for *n*=204 resulted in a mean of 0.6879, standard deviation of 0.117, and a 95% confidence interval of 0.67178, 0.70409. Results primarily followed the standard deviation, with additional clustering around the 75th and 85th percentiles. Normality was confirmed with an Anderson-Darling test of 0.440 and a P-value of 0.289 for the full population. Floor and ceiling effects were not encountered as no responses reached the lowest level, while only one response reached near the upper bound with a score of 0.9911.

In terms of construct validity, domain correlation shows relationships between the five Connor Davidson Resilience Scales (Vision, Composure, Reasoning, Tenacity, Collaboration) and the additional Health domain. The Composure and Reasoning domains displayed the strongest relationship, while relationships were also evident between the Connor Davidson Resilience Scale as is to be expected as part of traditional resilience factors. Pearson correlations between the additional Health domain and five Davidson scales were found to be positive at 0.169 with a p-value of 0.016. While the Pearson value in the lower range, the < 0.05 p-value result indicates the relation is of statistical significance. Item analysis yielded a Cronbach's α of 0.7364, indicating good internal consistency and validity as a psychometric tool.

With respect to scoring, raw score responses are added within each domain, and the raw score for all factors are added to achieve a total score. For the purpose of this study, the aim was to assess overall resilience globally. Thus, the analysis was based upon the total composite score.

Posttraumatic Growth Measure

The Posttraumatic Growth Inventory (PTGI; non-copyrighted), which was developed by Tedeschi and Calhoun in 1996, is one of the most widely used self-report measures to assess growth subsequent to trauma in adults (Gangstad et al., 2009). The measure consists of 21 items based upon a 6-point Likert scale: (0) I did not experience this change as a result of my crisis; (1) I experienced this change to a very small degree as a result of my crisis; (2) I experienced this change to a small degree as a result of my crisis; (3) I experienced this change to a moderate degree as a result of my crisis; (4) I experienced this change to a great degree as a result of my crisis; (5) I experienced this change to a very great degree as a result of my crisis. Raw scores range from 0 to 105 points. Higher scores reflect a higher PTG level. The scale includes 5 dimensions: relating to others, new possibilities, personal power, mental changes, and life enjoyment. Specific PTG questions were generated based upon the 3 main categories of perceived change in sense of self, interpersonal relationships, and philosophy on life. In terms of perceived change in sense of self, the authors posit that persons who work through a traumatic event draw the conclusion that they have developed mental fortitude, which they generalize to various situations moving forward. Change in interpersonal relationships is described as an enhanced willingness to express emotions, as well as increased sensitivity to the emotional needs of others. A nuanced philosophy on life is associated with an attempt to live life to its fullest. For instance, a study completed by Taylor et al. (1984) revealed that 60% of women with a breast cancer history endorsed positive changes in priorities, such as approaching life with more flexibility and savoring life's precious moments (Tedeschi & Calhoun, 1996). Review of the psychometric properties reveals internal consistency of the PTGI ($a = .90$), suggesting that items contribute relatively equally to consistency of scaled scores. Test-retest reliability ($r = .71$) was rated as acceptable.

A gender x severity of trauma multivariate analysis of variance with the five PTGI factors as dependent variables also demonstrated that women reported more benefits than did men $F(53,5) = 3.68, p < .01$, and persons experiencing severe trauma reported more benefits than those who did not $F(53,5) = 3.61$, $p < .01$ (Tedeschi & Calhoun, 1996). The gender x severity interaction was not significant, $F(53,5) = 1.36$. Univariate tests showed that women had higher scores than men for the New Possibilities factor, $F(1,113) = 6.15$, $p < .05$; the Relating to Others factor, $F(1,113) = 6.93$, $p < .01$; the Personal Strength factor, $F(1,113) = 4.96$, $p < .05$; and the Spiritual Change factor, $F(1,113) = 14.09$, $p < .001$, but not for the Appreciation of Life factor, $F(1,113) = 3.26$.

Data Collection Procedures

Prior to commencing actual data collection, I received approval from the Institutional Review Board (IRB) of Fielding Graduate University. This approval signified that the study adhered to appropriate ethical standards the institution has defined. After receiving ethical approval, I developed the survey on Qualtrics. The survey was comprised of a screening questionnaire, a consent form, a background information scale, and the main scales for assessing childhood abuse, resilience, and posttraumatic growth. I then drafted a recruitment letter and shared it alongside a link to the Qualtrics survey on different social media platforms, such as Facebook, Twitter, and LinkedIn. Interested participants used a link, which directed them to the first page of the survey containing the screening questionnaire and consent form. Participants were then prompted to respond to the screening questionnaire items. The purpose of the screening tool was to ensure only participants that met the inclusion criteria were actually recruited into the study.

Sampling

Convenience sampling was used to identify and select participants for inclusion in this study. Convenience sampling entailed identifying and recruiting participants based on the ease with which they can be accessed (Etikan et al., 2016). Considering that over 3.8 million women are breast cancer survivors, a convenience sample large enough for the current quantitative study was obtained easily. Using Qualtrics Survey, fraud detection, the data were screened for the robo/spam and multiple submissions.

Power Analysis for Sample Size Estimation

In determining an appropriate sample size for the current study, G*power analysis was conducted. The G*Power open-source software was used to determine an appropriate sample size. The analyses included both ANOVA-based analyses and regression-based analyses. A single-factor ANOVA (and ANCOVA) was used for H1 and H2. The analysis indicated a sample of $N = 159$ (ANOVA) or $N = 158$ (ANCOVA) would be required to detect moderate-sized effects ($f = .25$) with sufficient power (.80). The regression-based approach to mediation analysis relies on bias-corrected, bootstrapped confidence intervals to identify the significance of indirect (mediated) effects. Fritz and MacKinnon (2007) ran simulation analysis to determine sample size requirements for mediation models varying in the strength of the effects/association along the indirect path from predictor to mediator, and from mediator to outcome. The analysis indicated that required sample size ranged from $N = 462$ (if both effects along the indirect effect were small) to $N = 34$ (if both effects were large). With small to moderate effects along the indirect path (.26), a sample of $N = 148$ would be required. For the study, then, a sample of $N = 200$ was to be recruited, providing sufficient power for the ANOVA-based, and regression-based analyses. Participants who met the inclusion criteria as determined by the screening questionnaire were prompted to read and respond to the consent form. The consent form detailed information on the purpose of the study and an overview of the methods I used to collect data. The consent form specified that participating in the study was voluntary and that a participant would only get involved after signing the form. Participants who signed the consent form were directed to the second page of the survey containing items from the background information scale, physical and emotional abuse scale, resilience scale, and posttraumatic growth scale. Participants completed the questionnaires, and the information was automatically recorded in a spreadsheet. I then downloaded the spreadsheet onto my computer for data preparation and analysis.

This study used Qualtrics, an online survey and analytics company that provides the ability to design questionnaires and offers an online portal for potential survey respondents to access all of the measures used in this study in one convenient interaction. The separate measures are not delineated. Respondents' impression is that they are answering one survey, not a number of different measures.

The recruitment procedure included posting a link to social media platforms, such as Facebook, LinkedIn, Reddit, and Twitter. A link was posted in open group forums that invited participants to complete the survey. Closed groups had forum facilitators. The letter in Appendix A was sent to the facilitators asking for permission to post the link in their groups. There was no personal identifiable information (PIN), and therefore, participation was anonymous. For the purpose of organizing data, subject numbers were assigned to respective participants.

When initiating the survey, participants were prompted to review a description of the purpose of the study, as well as potential benefits and risks of participation. Participation signified informed consent. The consent form explicitly stated that participation was fully voluntary, and that participants could stop completing the survey/not submit responses at any time.

After informed consent, directions were offered. Based upon previous surveys, the completion time was estimated at 40 minutes. Participants completed the background questionnaire, Emotional and Physical Abuse Questionnaire (EPAB), The Symptom Checklist-90 Items (SCL-90), Predictive 6-Factor Resilience Scale (PR6), and Posttraumatic Growth Inventory (PTGI). After all data were collected, the data were first analyzed in Qualtrics native software. Then, the data were exported to SPSS for analysis. Data were password protected and could not be linked to any specific participant.

In terms of scoring, responses on the 6-point Likert scale were added to achieve a total raw score as well as raw score totals based on each of the 5 domains. For the purpose of this analysis, because posttraumatic growth was being assessed globally, only the total score was utilized.

Table 1

Summary of Control Variables

Variable	*Conceptual Definition*	*Measure/Operational Def.*	*Form of Data*	*Role*
Research-Defined Abuse	Used to refer to abusive experiences based upon research definitions	Emotional and Physical Abuse Questionnaire (EPAB): Physical Abuse (14 items) and Emotional Abuse (4 items)	Continuous (level of abuse): No Abuse; Mild Abuse: Severe Abuse; Ordinal: Level of Severity	DV: Predictor
Subjective Abuse	Subjective recall of abuse of physical and emotional abuse	Emotional and Physical Abuse Questionnaire (EPAB): Physical Abuse (1 item) and Emotional Abuse (1 item)	Nominal/Categorical	IV: Predictor
Resilience	Adaptation to Adverse Experience	Predictive 6-Factor Resilience Scale (PR6): 50-items; Composite Score	Interval	IV: Mediator & Outcome
Posttraumatic Growth	Personal Growth in response to Adverse Experiences	Posttraumatic Growth Inventory (PTGI): 21 items; Composite Score	Interval	Outcome

The bivariate association between the demographic variables (mental health history, alcohol history, age, ethnicity, income, level of education, religiosity) and the primary outcome (posttraumatic growth) were examined. Those demographic variables that were significantly associated with the outcome were treated as covariates in subsequent analyses pertaining to the four hypotheses. For each hypothesis, then, an unadjusted (w/o covariates) and an adjusted (with covariates) model were run.

CHAPTER FIVE: RESULTS

This study examined the impact of early physical and emotional abuse during childhood on resilience and posttraumatic growth following breast cancer survival. The previous chapter included a discussion of the methods used to collect and analyze data in this study. This chapter focuses on the presentation of the findings obtained after the data were collected and analyzed. The chapter begins with a review of the preliminary analysis and data screening conducted. The next subsection contains the descriptive statistics of the different variables of interest in the study. Lastly, results obtained from inferential statistical analyses are presented, and the four hypotheses under the main research question in this study are tested. The chapter concludes with a summary and transitions to the next chapter.

Preliminary Analysis

The response data from Qualtrics were imported into the data editor of IBM SPSS Statistics 27.0. The responses to The Background Questionnaire, Emotional and Physical Abuse Questionnaire (EPAB), the Symptom Checklist-90 items (SCL-90; non-copyrighted version), the Predictive 6-Factor Resilience Scale (PR6), the Posttraumatic Growth Inventory (PTGI), the Research and Development (RAND) 36-Item Short Form Health Survey (SF-36), and the BREAST-Q 2 were screened and cleaned. Five hundred twenty-three respondents participated in the survey. Four participants were excluded because they had no history of breast cancer (N = 519). Seventy-six participants were excluded because they had no history of breast cancer treatment (N = 443). One hundred twenty-nine were excluded because they were not diagnosed with breast cancer in the past 2 years (N = 314). One participant was excluded due to being younger than 18 years of age (N = 313). Seven male participants were excluded because this study examined female experiences (N = 306). One hundred nineteen participants were excluded because they contained missing data. Thus, the total number of participants after screening and cleaning was 187.

Data Screening

Before analyses, data from the PR6 (total and subscales) and PTGI were screened for distributional assumptions and outliers. All distributions were effectively normal, as skewness and kurtosis values fell between +/-1.0. While some outliers were identified on the resilience measures (total scores and vision, composure, and reasoning subscales), they were found at both the low and high ends of the distributions, which were otherwise normal in shape. For this reason, the outlying cases were retained in subsequent analyses.

Table 2 presents descriptive statistics on the PTGI, Resilience, Breast Cancer Quality of Life (QOL; well-being, worry), and the RAND scales. Means on the total scores and subscales were comparable to those reported for the normative samples used in developing these instruments (Klassen et al., 2021; Ware & Sherbourne, 1992). Review of mean RAND scores reveals a greater perceived limitation in terms of physical role functioning, emotional role functioning in breast cancer survivors. Review of the skewness and kurtosis values serves as evidence that the distributions were effectively normal with the exception of the RAND scales, which were slightly platykurtic. Although variability was high, the RAND scales were balanced/symmetrical. No outliers were detected on the RAND scales.

Table 2

Distributional Assumptions for Core Variables

Variable Name	*N*	*M*	*SD*	Skewness	Kurtosis
PTGI Total	187	49.8556	24.50818	-.376	-.582
PR-Tenacity	182	.6984	.18611	-.277	-.226
PR-Momentum	186	.6597	.18406	-.221	-.064
Total Resilience	187	.6442	.13781	-.342	.932
BC QOL Well-Being	186	54.7419	19.10902	.099	.620
BC Worry	185	56.1459	17.49147	.519	.803
RAND Physical Limitations	185	43.6486	42.87000	.297	-1.650
RAND Emotional Limitations	185	46.6667	43.43355	.162	-1.708
Perceptions of General Health	184	47.5996	24.25564	.019	-1.040

Descriptive Statistics of Participants

The demographic characteristics of the 187 participants were analyzed. Table 3 outlines the sample's demographic characteristics in general, while Table 4 summarizes the demographic characteristics of participants' breast cancer experience. Participants' ages ranged from 18-24 through 66+ years. The most frequent age range was from 35-44 (28.3%), followed by the age range 55-65 (23%), ages 25-34 (20.3%), ages 45-54 (16%), ages 66+ (11.2%), and ages 18-24 (1.1%). The distribution of ages is suggestive that persons in the 66+ age category were less likely to complete surveys on an online forum. Further, women of the ages of 18-24 were less likely to be diagnosed with breast cancer, and they were less likely to be 2 plus years out from a breast cancer diagnosis. In terms of educational attainment, the most frequent level of education was an undergraduate school/bachelor's degree (32.1%), followed by community college/technical school/associate degree (28.9%), high school education (26.2%), graduate school (master's, PhD, MD; 11.2%), and middle school (1.6%). Half of the sample identified as White (50.3%), followed by Black/African American/African Origins (17.1%), Latino-a/Hispanic (12.8%), Asian American/Asian Origin/ Pacific Islander (9.1%), Native American Indian/Alaska Native/Aboriginal (6.4%), Biracial/Multi-Racial (2.1%), and Other (.5%). Overall, ethnicity was balanced as compared to the United States population as a whole.

Table 3

Demographic Characteristic of Sample (N = 187)

Characteristics	Category	*n*	%
Age	18-24	2	1.1
	25-34	38	20.3
	35-44	53	28.3
	45-54	30	16.0
	55-65	43	23.0
	66+	21	11.2
Education	Middle School (6-8)	3	1.6
	High School (9-12)	49	26.2
	Community College/Technical School/Associate degree	54	28.9
	Undergraduate School (Bachelor's degree)	60	32.1
	Graduate School (Master's, PhD, MD)	21	11.2
Employment	Farm laborer, day laborer	4	2.1
	Unskilled worker, service worker	11	5.9
	Machine operator, semiskilled worker	15	8.0
	Skilled manual worker, craftsman, police and fire services, enlisted military	9	4.8
	Clerical/sales, small farm owner	5	2.7
	Technicians, semiprofessional, supervisor, office manager	30	16.0
	Professional, technical, and managerial occupations	48	25.7
	Miscellaneous	45	24.1
Income	Less than $25,000	8	4.3
	$25,000-$49,999	31	16.6
	$50,000-$74,999	55	29.4
	$75,000-$99,999	49	26.2
	$100,000-$149,999	24	12.8
	$150,000 or more	16	8.6
	Prefer not to say	4	2.1
Ethnicity	Black/African American/African Origins	32	17.1
	Asian American/Asian Origin/ Pacific Islander	17	9.1
	Latino-a/ Hispanic	24	12.8
	Native American Indian/Alaska Native/Aboriginal	12	6.4
	White/European Origin	94	50.3

Characteristics	Category	*n*	%
	Bi-racial /multi-racial	4	2.1
	Other	1	.5
Relationship status	Married	148	79.1
	Living with a partner	26	6
	Never married	6	3.2
	Widowed	13	7
	Separated	4	2.1
	Divorced	23	12.3
	Divorced x1	13	7
	Divorced x2	6	3.2
	Divorced x3	1	.5
	Divorced x4	1	.5
Gender	Female	186	99.5
	Nonbinary	1	.5
Cancer Stages	Stage 0		5.17
	Stage 1		23.99
	Stage 2		44.28
	Stage 3		22.88
	Stage 4		3.69
Years of Survival	2 to 5 years		45.58
	6 to 10 years		18.60
	11 to 15 years		14.42
	16 to 20 years		12.09
	Over 20 years		9.30

Table 4 outlines characteristics specific to participants' cancer experience. The most frequent response in terms of breast cancer stage at the time of diagnosis was Stage 2 (41.2%), followed by Stage 3 (27.8%), Stage 1 (23.5%), Stage 4 (4.3%), and Stage 0 (3.2%). The lowest area of response was for women with Stage 0 breast cancer. It is reasonable that persons with Stage 0 breast cancer may not perceive themselves to be breast cancer survivors. The second lowest group response was with Stage 4 breast cancer, which is reasonable considering the level of mortality associated with a Stage 4 diagnosis. The majority of responses were with stages 2 and 3, which is consistent with the aim of this study in terms of examining the long-term experiences of breast cancer survivors. Regarding the number of years since diagnosis, the most frequent response was 2 to 5 years (36.9%), followed by 6 to 10 years (14.4%), 16 to 20 years (12.8%), over 20 years (9.1%), and 11 to 15 years (7.5%). Over one-third of participants reported metastatic disease secondary to breast cancer (35.3%). Almost half of the participants experienced breast cancer recurrence (44.4%). Slightly more than one-fourth of participants suffered additional cancer (other than breast cancer) that required medical treatment (26.2%). The study also includes ethnically diverse subjects, which is in line with the United States Census of 2020. The ethnic characteristics include White/European Origin (50.3%), Black/African American/African Origins (17.1%), Latino-a / Hispanic (12.8%), Asian American/Asian Origin/ Pacific Islander (9.1%), Native American Indian/Alaska Native/Aboriginal (6.4%), Bi-racial /multi-Racial (2.1%), and Other (.5%).

Table 4

Breast Cancer Characteristics of Sample (N = 187)

Characteristics	Category	*n*	%
Stage at diagnosis	Stage 0	6	3.2
	Stage 1	44	23.5
	Stage 2	77	41.2
	Stage 3	52	27.8
	Stage 4	8	4.3
Years of survival	2 to 5 years	69	36.9
	6 to 10 years	27	14.4
	11 to 15 years	14	7.5
	16 to 20 years	24	12.8
	Over 20 years	17	9.1
Additional cancer	Metastatic breast cancer	66	35.3
	Breast cancer recurrence	83	44.4
	Additional cancer that required treatment	49	26.2
Decreased body image (present)	Not at all	38	20.3
	Slightly true	55	29.4
	True	46	24.6
	Mostly true	29	15.5
	Very True	19	10.2
More spiritual	Not at all	49	26.2
	Slightly true	60	32.1
	True	49	26.2
	Mostly true	17	9.1
	Very true	11	5.9
More religious	Not at all	40	21.4
	Slightly true	45	24.1
	True	62	33.2
	Mostly true	28	15.0
	Very true	12	6.4
Mental health treatment	Therapy prior to breast cancer	93	49.7
	Therapy during breast cancer	104	55.6
	Therapy after breast cancer	117	62.6
	History of psychiatric hospitalization	58	31.0
Financial burden (current)	Not at all	67	35.8
	Slightly true	45	24.1
	True	34	18.2
	Mostly true	25	13.4
	Very True	16	8.6

Descriptive Statistics of the Abuse Measure

A descriptive analysis of the variables was completed. This analysis included frequency distributions, percentages, means, and standard deviations. This section presents the descriptive statistics of the variables.

The first analysis examined physical abuse severity based on researcher-defined abuse. The EPAB items are on a 6-point Likert scale (0 = *Never* to 5 = *Very Frequently),* and overall participant responses indicate no abuse, mild abuse, or abused (severe). Participants were coded as "mild abuse" if they endorsed any frequency of the following three items: "I was spanked or hit," "I was pinched as punishment," or "I was hit or spanked with a belt." Participants were coded as having been "abused" if they rated any of the nine major assault questions on the EPAB with a frequency of 1 or greater than the nine assault items. The nine assault items are as follows: 1-"I have received black eyes from being hit"; 2-"Thrown against the wall"; 3-"I was injured seriously enough by a parent or guardian to require medical care"; 4-"I have had broken bones following a beating"; 5- "I was purposefully burned with a cigarette lighter, iron, etc."; 6-"I was bitten so hard marks were left, or my skin was broken"; 7- "I have had teeth loosened or knocked out"; 8-"My hair was snatched or pulled out"; 9- "I was strangled or choked." Participants were also coded as "abused" if they rated five items that are not major assault items with a frequency of 3 or greater ("I was pinched as punishment," "I was hit or spanked with a board, stick, or wire," "I was tied up as punishment," "I was hit or spanked with a belt," "I was shaken"). All other participants were coded as "not abused."

The descriptive analysis of the physical abuse variable is outlined in Table 5. Most participants endorsed items that are consistent with severe abuse (70.4%), followed by mild abuse (17.2%), and no physical abuse (12.4%). Overall results reveal a higher level of physical abuse in the current breast cancer population, as compared to a general/adult population (Wolkins, 2020). Previous results of the EPAB physical abuse in a general population measure revealed severe abuse (33%), mild abuse (54%), and no abuse (12.6%; Wolkins, 2020). Thus, although researcher-defined abuse was similar for the no abuse category, severe abuse was significantly higher in the current population.

Table 5

Physical Abuse Severity (N = 186)

Researcher-defined abuse	*N*	%
No physical abuse	23	12.4
Mild physical abuse	32	17.2
Physical abuse (severe)	131	70.4

Emotional abuse on the EPAB comprises four items rated on a 6-point Likert-type scale (0 = *never* to 5 = *very frequently*). Items include (1) “I was mocked or taunted,” (2) “I was ridiculed in front of friends or strangers,” (3) “At home I was criticized and made to feel worthless,” and (4) “I saw other family members humiliated.” My definition of the frequency of childhood emotional abuse variable was calculated by averaging the responses of the four items. Thus, descriptive analysis of emotional abuse was based on mean responses.

The descriptive analysis of the emotional abuse variable is outlined. The average score for the 187 participants in terms of emotional abuse was 1.844 (SD = 1.383). This sample of female survivors of breast cancer reported significantly higher levels of emotional abuse as compared to a general, adult population (M = 1.84, SD = 1.38) than levels of emotional abuse previously reported (M = 1.06, SD = 1.31 . . t (186) = 7.75, $p < .001$; Wolkins, 2020).

Table 6

Mean Responses to Emotional Abuse Items (N = 187)

Research-defined abuse	*n*	*M*	SD
Emotional Abuse	187	1.844	1.383

Covariates

The association between demographic characteristics (age, ethnicity, stage of cancer, cancer recurrence, substance abuse, and therapy before, during, and after diagnosis) and the outcome of interest, posttraumatic growth, were all non-significant. There was no need, therefore, to treat any of these factors as covariates in subsequent analyses. However, associations between scores on the Breast Cancer QOL, well-being and worry scales and the RAND physical limitations, limitations due to emotional/personal problems, and perceptions of general health were significantly associated with posttraumatic growth (see Table 7). As seen in this table, on the Breast Cancer QOL measure, well-being was positively associated with PTGI total scores ($r = .354$), and worry was negatively associated with this outcome ($r = -.282$). On the RAND, perceptions of physical limitations, perception of emotional limitations, and perceptions of general health were analyzed concerning total PTGI. Lack of physical limitations was positively associated with PTGI total scores ($r = .311$). Lack of emotional limitations regarding role fulfillment was positively associated with PTGI total scores ($r = .306$). Perceptions of favorable health, in general, were positively associated with PTGI total scores ($r = .279$). Scores deriving from these five scales were thus included as covariates in subsequent analyses. All scales BC QOL Well-Being; BC Worry; RAND Physical Limits; RAND Emotional Limits, and RAND Perceptions of General Health were significantly correlated with the posttraumatic growth outcome. Please note that negative values with RAND Physical Limits and RAND

Emotional Limits were positively associated with BC Worry. That is, the greater the perceived physical and emotional limits, the greater breast cancer worry. Conversely, positive values for RAND Physical Limits and RAND Emotional Limits were both positively associated with RAND Perceptions of General Health. Specifically, less perceived physical and emotional limitations were associated with perceptions of favorable general health.

Table 7

Bivariate Correlations between Breast Cancer Well-Being and Worry, RAND Scales, and PTGI

	PTGI Total	BC QOL Well-Being	BC Worry	RAND Physical Limits	RAND Emotional Limits	RAND General Health Perceptions
PTGI Total	1.000					
BC QOL Well-Being	.354	1.000				
BC Worry	-.282	-.409**	1.000			
RAND Physical Limits	.311	.450**	-.413**	1.000		
RAND Emotional Limits	.306	.507**	-.434**	.774**	1.000	
RAND Perceptions of General Health	.279	.558**	-.600**	.570**	.606**	1.000

**. Correlation is significant at the 0.01 level (2-tailed).

Bivariate correlations between all the variables under consideration can be found in Table 8. As seen in this table, there was no (unadjusted) association between posttraumatic growth and the abuse measures. There were, however, significant associations between resilience and posttraumatic growth, as well as between what served as the covariates in subsequent analyses (see Table 7) and posttraumatic growth. Of all the bivariate correlations, the strongest was between resilience and posttraumatic growth. Further mild physical abuse was positively associated with resilience, while severe physical abuse was negatively associated with resilience.

Table 8

Correlation Matrix Including all Variables: Emotional Abuse (EA), Mild Physical Abuse (PA), Severe PA, Resilience, Posttraumatic Growth, Breast Cancer Quality of Life (BC QOL) Well-Being, BC Worry, and RAND Scales Including Perceptions of General Health, Emotional Personal Limitations, and Limitations due to Physical Health

	PTGI Total	Mean EA	Mild PA	Severe PA	Total Resili-ence	BC QOL Well-Being	BC Worry	RAND General Health	RAND Emo-tional Limita-tions	RA Phy Lim tic
PTGI Total	1.000									
Mean EA	-.007	1.000								
Mild PA	.022	-.287**	1.000							
Severe PA	.037	.578**	-.704**	1.000						
Total Resilience	.492**	-.372**	.243**	-.366**	1.000					
BC QOL Well-Being	.354**	-.374**	.219**	-.421**	.650**	1.000				
BC Worry	-.282**	.274**	-.165*	.262**	-.507**	-.409**	1.000			
RAND General Health	.279**	-.258**	.119	-.295**	.622**	.558**	-.600**	1.000		
RAND Emot. Limit	.306**	-.306**	.233**	-.445**	.541**	.507**	-.434**	.606**	1.000	
RAND Physical Limit	.309**	-.193	.109	-.338**	.538**	.429**	-.407**	.582**	.783**	1.

**. Correlation is significant at the 0.01 level (2-tailed).
*. Correlation is significant at the 0.05 level (2-tailed).

H_1 Hypothesis 1

The first hypothesis concerned the association between emotional abuse, physical abuse, and posttraumatic growth. To test this first hypothesis, two hierarchical regression analyses were conducted. The first hierarchical regression was intended to test whether emotional abuse was significantly associated with posttraumatic growth. In this first hierarchical regression analysis, the covariates BC QOL Well-Being, BC Worry, RAND Physical Limitations, RAND Emotional Limitations, and RAND Perception of General Health were entered in the first step, and the predictor of interest (emotional abuse, physical abuse severity) was entered in a second step. Emotional abuse was found to be significantly associated with posttraumatic growth as indicated by the significant R-squared change when this predictor of interest was added to the model in the second step $\Delta R^2 = .025$, $F_{chg}\ (1, 177) = 5.52$, $p = .02$ (Table 9). The findings indicate that emotional abuse accounted for 2.5% of all variation in posttraumatic growth.

Table 9

Model Summary of Emotional Abuse as a Predictor of Posttraumatic Growth

Model	R	R^2	R_{2adj}	ΔR^2	F_{chg}	p	df_1	df_2
1	.405	.164	.141	.164	6.993	.000	5	178
2	.435	.189	.162	.025	5.52	.020	1	177

As shown in the regression coefficients table (Table 10), emotional abuse was positively associated with posttraumatic growth (β = .175, p = 0.020). As such, higher levels of emotional abuse corresponded with higher levels of posttraumatic growth. Of the covariates in the model, only BC QOL well-being was also positively associated with posttraumatic growth (β = .277, p = 0.002). None of the other covariates were significantly associated with posttraumatic growth in the adjusted model.

Table 10

Emotional Abuse as a Predictor of Posttraumatic Growth

	B	*S.E.*	*β*	*T*	*P*
(Constant)	34.483	11.219		3.074	.002
BC QOL Well-Being	.353	.112	.277	3.168	.002
BC Worry	-.221	.120	-.158	-1.836	.068
RAND Physical Limitations	.081	.082	.110	.994	.322
RAND Emotional Limitations	.053	.066	.094	.807	.421
Perception of General Health	-.046	.103	-.045	-.444	.657
Emotional Abuse Items	3.071	1.307	.175	2.349	.020

The second hierarchical regression model included physical abuse as the key variable of interest. Similar to the first hierarchical regression, the covariates entered in the first step were BC QOL Well-Being, BC Worry, RAND Physical Limitations, RAND Emotional Limitations, and RAND Perception of General Health. The change statistic indicated that physical abuse severity contributed significantly to the model predicting posttraumatic growth, R^2 Change = .093, F (2, 175) = 10.99, p <.001. See table 11. In other words, more severe physical abuse tended to be associated with higher levels of posttraumatic growth.

Table 11

Model Summary: Physical Abuse as a Predictor of Posttraumatic Growth

Model	R	R^2	R_{2adj}	ΔR^2	F_{chg}	p	df_1	df_2
1	.403	.162	.139	.162	6.854	.000	5	177
2	.506	.256	.226	.093	10.985	.000	2	175

Coefficients from the physical abuse final (Step 2) adjusted model can be found in Table 12. Both mild (β = .206, p = 0.030) and severe (β = 0.468, p < .001) physical abuse were positively associated with posttraumatic growth. The findings suggest that compared to no abuse, persons who suffered mild physical abuse were more likely to experience posttraumatic growth. Similarly, persons who experienced severe physical abuse were more likely than those who experienced no abuse to develop posttraumatic growth. Of all the covariates included in the model, only Perception of General Health had a significant positive association with posttraumatic growth (B = 13.112, p = 0.03).

Table 12

Mild Physical Abuse and Severe Physical Abuse as Predictors of Posttraumatic Growth

	B	*S.E.*	*β*	*T*	*P*
(Constant)	14.638	12.198	-	1.200	.232
BC QOL Well-Being	.405	.108	.318	3.758	.000*
BC Worry	-.202	.114	-.146	-1.764	.080
RAND Physical Limitations	.091	.062	.161	1.460	.146
RAND Emotional Limitations	.083	.066	.149	1,269	.206
Perception of General Health	-.055	.099	-.055	-.552	.582
Mild PA	13.112	5.989	.206	2.189	.030*
Severe PA	24.73	5.740	.468	4.520	.000*

H_2 Hypothesis 2

The second hypothesis examined the association between abuse and resilience. In referring to the overall correlation matrix as outlined above in Table 8, emotional abuse was negatively associated with resilience overall ($R = -.372$), mild physical abuse was positively associated with resilience ($R = .243$), and severe physical abuse was negatively associated ($R = -.366$). These unadjusted associations were further examined in hierarchical regression models. The abuse measures were added in a second step to models including the covariates (BC QOL Well-Being, BC Worry, RAND Physical Limitations, RAND Emotional Limitations, and RAND Perception of General Health).

Two hierarchical regression models were run to determine whether emotional and physical abuse were significantly associated with resilience. In the first model, emotional abuse was the key variable of interest. The first step included only the covariates BC QOL Well-Being, BC Worry, RAND Physical Limitations, RAND Emotional Limitations, and RAND Perception of General Health. In the second step, emotional abuse was added to the list of predictors as a variable of interest. Table 13 contains the hierarchical regression results for emotional abuse. As shown in the table, adding emotional abuse resulted in a significant increase in the explained variance $\Delta R^2 = .0.011$, $F_{chgf}(1, 177) = 4.488$, $p = .036$ (Table 13). Thus, emotional abuse alone accounted for 1.1% of all variations in resilience.

Table 13

Model Summary of Hierarchical Regression for Emotional Abuse

Model	R	R^2	R_{2adj}	ΔR^2	F_{chg}	p	df_1	df_2
1	.748	.560	.548	.560	45.350	.000	5	178
2	.756	.571	.557	.011	4.488	.036	1	177

Table 14 contains the regression coefficients for the analysis conducted. Emotional abuse was positively associated with resilience (B = 0.003, $p = 0.00$). Based upon the positive relationship of change with the regression coefficient, as the independent variable increases (emotional abuse), the dependent variable also increases (resilience). The findings indicate that persons who experienced higher levels of emotional abuse were more likely to develop resilience than those who experienced a lower degree of emotional abuse. The following covariates in the model were also significantly associated with resilience: BC QOL Well-Being (B = -0.001, $p = 0.038$), BC Worry (B = 0.001, $p = 0.007$), RAND Emotional Limitations (B = 0.001, $p = 0.019$), and Perception of General Health (B = -0.011, $p = 0.036$).

Table 14

Emotional Abuse as a Predictor of Resilience

	B	*S.E.*	*β*	*t*	*p*
(Constant)	.003	.000	.361	5.670	.000
BC QOL Well-Being	-.001	.000	-.131	-2.096	.038
BC Worry	.001	.000	.204	2.739	.007
RAND Physical Limitations	-3.297	.000	-.010	-.118	.906
RAND Emotional Limitations	.001	.000	.196	2.363	.019
Perception of General Health	-.011	.005	-.115	-2.118	.036
Mean Response to Emotional Abuse Items	.003	.000	.361	5.670	.000

In the second hierarchical regression model, physical abuse was the key variable of interest. A similar analysis to the first hierarchical regression model was conducted but with physical abuse as the predictor of interest this time. The results of the hierarchical regression analysis are shown in Table 15. Physical abuse was associated with resilience, although the amount of explained variance was not significant, as shown by the non-significant R-squared change, $\Delta R^2 = .0.009$, F_{chg} (2, 175) = 1.792, $p = .170$ (Table 15). The R-squared change indicates that the explained variance in resilience improved by 0.9% when physical abuse was included in the model.

Table 15

Model Summary of Hierarchical Regression for Physical Abuse

Model	R	R^2	R_{2adj}	ΔR^2	F_{chg}	p	df_1	df_2
1	.749	.560	.548	.560	45.121	.000	5	177
2	.754	.569	.557	.009	1.792	.170	2	175

Table 16 contains regression coefficients for the model covariates and physical abuse. Mild physical abuse was not significantly associated with resilience (B = 0.045, p = 0.089). Severe physical abuse was also not significantly associated with resilience (B = 0.014, p = 0.564). The following covariates were significantly associated with resilience: BC QOL Well-Being (B = 0.003, p = 0.000), BC Worry (B = -0.001, p = 0.031), RAND Physical Limitations (B = 0.001, p = 0.007), and Perception of General Health (B = 0.001, p = 0.018). As predicted, although nonsignificant, mild abuse, as opposed to severe abuse, is associated with posttraumatic growth, and resilience is a mediator of posttraumatic growth.

Table 16

Mild Physical Abuse and Severe Physical Abuse as Predictors of Resilience

	B	*S.E.*	*β*	*t*	*p*
(Constant)	.449	.053		8.443	.000
BC QOL Well-Being	.003	.000	.388	6.020	.000
BC Worry	-.001	.000	-.137	-2.170	.031
RAND Physical Limitations	.001	.000	.208	2.752	.034
RAND Emotional Limitations	-1.721E-5	.000	-.005	-.060	.834
Perception of General Health	.001	.000	.200	2.385	.007
Mild PA	.045	.026	.122	1.710	.089
Severe PA	.014	.024	.046	.578	.564

H_3 Hypothesis 3

The third hypothesis examined whether resilience would be positively associated with posttraumatic growth. A hierarchical regression analysis was conducted to determine whether resilience was significantly associated with posttraumatic growth. In the first step, only the covariates were entered. In the second step, resilience was added as the variable of interest. The results of the analysis are shown in Table 17. Resilience was significantly associated with posttraumatic growth, as indicated by the significant R-squared change, $\Delta R^2 = .0.089$, F_{chg} (1, 177) = 21.175, $p = .000$ (Tale 17). Thus, adding resilience to the regression model improved explained variation in posttraumatic growth by 8.9%.

Table 17

Model Summary of Relationship Between Resilience and Posttraumatic Growth

Model	R	R^2	R_{2adj}	ΔR^2	F_{chg}	*p*	df_1	df_2
1	.406	.165	.165	.165	7.038	.000	5	178
2	.504	.254	.229	.089	21.175	.000	1	177

Table 18 contains the regression coefficients for the hierarchical regression model. Resilience was positively associated with posttraumatic growth (B = 79.216, p = 0.00). Thus, persons with greater resilience levels were likely to develop posttraumatic growth. None of the covariates in the model were significantly associated with posttraumatic growth.

Table 18

Hierarchical Regression for Relationship Between Resilience and Posttraumatic Growth

	B	S.E.	β	T	p
(Constant)	4.467	13.144		.340	.734
BC QOL Well-Being	.070	.115	.055	.611	.542
BC Worry	-.096	.116	-.069	-.828	.409
RAND Physical Limitations	-.132	.101	-.131	-1.307	.193
RAND Emotional Limitations	.021	.064	.038	.331	.741
Perception of General Health	.034	.063	.060	.549	.584
Total Resilience	79.216	17.215	.450	4.602	.000

H_4 Hypothesis 4

Resilience Mediates Effects of Emotional Abuse on Posttraumatic Growth

The mediating effects of resilience were tested with a regression-based approach using the PROCESS software (Hayes, 2018). Evidence of mediation takes the form of a significant indirect effect indicated by bias-corrected bootstrapped confidence intervals excluding zero effect. The upper and lower limits are both positive or negative when there is a significant indirect effect. The first mediation analysis tested whether resilience mediated the effects of emotional abuse on posttraumatic growth. As before, the covariates were included in each mediation model tested. A path diagram depicting the results of this analysis can be found in Figure 2. As seen in the diagram, the association between emotional abuse and resilience and between resilience and posttraumatic growth were significant, yielding a significant indirect effect = -.954 (-2.05, -.08) In other words, the association between emotional abuse and posttraumatic growth can be explained, at least in part, by the association between emotional abuse and resilience which, in turn, had a direct effect on posttraumatic growth.

Figure 2

Mediation Analysis of Emotional Abuse and Resilience and Direct Effect on Posttraumatic Growth

Note: The diagram includes unstandardized regression coefficients with standardized coefficients in parentheses.

Resilience Mediates Effects of Physical Abuse on Posttraumatic Growth

A second mediation model was tested where PA severity was treated as the predictor of PTG. Results of this analysis are presented in Figure 3. Neither mild PA 3.62 (-.88, 9.27) or severe PA 1.12 (-2.93, 6.45) had significant indirect effects on PTG. As seen in Figure 2, this appeared to be due to the fact that neither predictor was significantly associated with the mediator (resilience). While PA severity was not sig associated with resilience, 4 of the 5 covariates (BC well-being, BC worry, General health, and physical health limitations) were associated with resilience (emotional health limitations were not). In the full adjusted model (that included PA severity, resilience, and the five covariates), only severe PA and resilience had sig direct effects on PTG (see path diagram).

Figure 3

Mediation Analysis of Physical Abuse Severity and Resilience and Effect on Posttraumatic Growth

CHAPTER SIX: DISCUSSION

This study examined the impact of early physical and emotional abuse during childhood on resilience and posttraumatic growth following breast cancer survival. Resilience and posttraumatic growth both refer to strength in meeting life's challenges; however, resilience and posttraumatic growth are two distinct constructs. Resilience is described as multifaceted adaption to adversity and the ability to access and utilize resources when confronted with traumatic events (Schulz et al., 2014). Resilience is considered a dynamic personality trait that is flexible, allowing persons to react to adversity. While resilience relates to adapting to adversity, posttraumatic growth refers to the psychological moving beyond pre-trauma levels of adaptation (Mohr & Rosén, 2017). Posttraumatic growth is defined as the positive psychological changes that one experiences after a stressful or traumatic event (Maitlis, 2020).

Numerous studies (Adams et al., 2018; Berger et al., 2015; Bretherton, 1992) have found that both childhood physical and emotional abuse are associated with lifelong mental health dysfunction; however, some research (Schaefer et al., 2018; Tranter et al., 2020; Tedeschi et al., 2018; Maitlis, 2020) has established that persons who adapt to unfavorable circumstances are more amenable to developing growth when confronting future challenges. This addressed a gap in the literature, exploring whether resilience and growth experienced from childhood trauma would aid in developing positive long-term adjustment to the emotional trauma of breast cancer. This study examined the relationship between resilience and posttraumatic growth and childhood abuse experiences in breast cancer survivors. To understand whether some types of early life abusive experiences yield resilience and posttraumatic growth, this investigation utilized measures of retrospective report of abusive conditions based upon research-defined abuse in relation to measures of resilience and posttraumatic growth. The aim of this study was to understand whether physical abuse severity or emotional abuse severity would impact resilience and posttraumatic growth in women who have survived breast cancer for 2 or more years.

Hypothesis 1

Hypothesis 1 posited that mild physical/emotional abuse during childhood would be associated with greater levels of posttraumatic growth than would either no abuse or more severe levels of abuse. In partial support of this hypothesis, physical abuse severity contributed significantly to predicting posttraumatic growth. While Hypothesis 1 predicted that (only) mild as opposed to severe physical abuse would predict posttraumatic growth, results revealed that both mild and severe physical abuse were significantly positively associated with posttraumatic growth. Although not statistically different, severe physical abuse was more positively associated with posttraumatic growth than mild physical abuse. Findings suggest that subjects who suffered either mild or severe physical abuse were more likely to experience posttraumatic growth, as compared to those in the no abuse category.

These findings suggest that physically abusive experiences in childhood may result in greater levels of growth when adapting to adverse events in adulthood, such as breast cancer. This is consistent with an assumption of posttraumatic growth theory in that more extreme events may produce more positive change as compared to less challenging circumstances (Tedeschi & Calhoun, 1996). Further, breast cancer survivors who experienced physical abuse in childhood and who possess a greater degree of psychosocial well-being, such as feeling confident, accepting of body image, feeling feminine in clothing, and so forth, tended to appreciate a greater degree of posttraumatic growth versus survivors who possess poor perceptions of general health, those who view themselves as emotionally unhealthy, and those who report that they possess physical limitations. Current findings are consistent with the prior research of Costanzo et al. (2009) who determined that in the long term, cancer survivors tend to experience greater degrees of personal growth as compared to healthy controls.

Also related to the physical abuse aspect of Hypothesis 1, current results of breast cancer survivors are in contrast with previous results within a general population. Previous results of the EPAB physical abuse measure revealed severe abuse (33%), mild abuse (54%), and no abuse (12.6%; Wolkins, 2020). This contrasts with EPAB physical abuse severity in the current study, which showed severe abuse (70.4%), mild abuse (17.2%), and no abuse (12.4%). While the proportion of adults within the no abuse category is relatively the same between both samples, the current study reveals a sample of women with a greater level of severe abuse and a lower level of mild abuse. Although not central to this study, the current results reveal a greater report of severe childhood physical abuse in breast cancer survivors as opposed to a general population. Findings of Hovdestad et al. (2020) indicated that of all forms of abuse, physical abuse was most highly associated with a cancer diagnosis. The same study revealed that with greater frequency and severity of childhood physical abuse, there was an increase in cancer diagnoses specifically in women. The current study further substantiates previous findings.

Similar to the physical abuse results, the study revealed that emotional abuse was positively associated with posttraumatic growth, indicating that with higher levels of emotional abuse, more posttraumatic growth occurred. While higher levels of emotional abuse in childhood were associated with more posttraumatic growth in breast cancer survivors, the scoring method of the measure used for emotional abuse (EPAB) did not provide the mild and severe categories that were delineated in scoring of physical abuse. Within the emotional abuse category, breast cancer survivors who possessed an overall sense of psychosocial well-being, such as feeling confident, accepting of body image, feeling feminine in clothing, and so forth, tended to appreciate a greater degree of posttraumatic growth versus survivors who possess poor perceptions of general health, those who view themselves as emotionally unhealthy, and those who report that they possess physical limitations. The current findings are in line with previous research in that favorable self-esteem is associated with posttraumatic growth.

Hypothesis 2

Hypothesis 2 suggested that mild physical/emotional abuse will be associated with greater levels of resilience than either no abuse or more severe levels of abuse. When examining emotional and physical abuse in relation to resilience, without controlling for other factors, emotional abuse was negatively associated, mild physical abuse was positively associated, and severe physical abuse was negatively associated with resilience.

Hypothesis 2, Emotional Abuse

Although emotional abuse was not positively associated with resilience in the initial analysis, there was a significant association between emotional abuse and resilience when breast cancer survivors endorsed favorable psychosocial well-being, low levels of worry regarding health factors associated with breast cancer, non-significant emotional limitations, and a favorable perception of their general health. Specifically, higher levels of emotional abuse were associated with higher levels of resilience when controlling for the preceding wellbeing factors. Essentially, breast cancer survivors who sustained emotional abuse during childhood showed greater resilience when they believed they were not negatively impacted by their breast cancer experience (either physically and/or emotionally) in the long term. Current findings are consistent with Martínez-Martí and Ruch (2017), who found that persons who suffered physical illness and who considered themselves resilient tended to show positive affect, self-efficacy, optimism, social support, self-esteem, and life satisfaction, independent of socioeconomic factors. Furthermore, Schulz et al. (2014) offered the notion that resilience is a skillful and multifaceted means of adaptation to adversity. Considering this, a potential explanation for the positive relationship between emotional abuse, resilience, and favorable perception of quality of life is that resilient survivors may better show positive affect, self-efficacy, optimism, social support, self-esteem, and life satisfaction. This is due to the fact that breast cancer survivors have further refined their innate resilience due to their history of emotional abuse.

Hypothesis 2, Physical Abuse

As expected, mild but not severe physical abuse was significantly associated with resilience within the straightforward analysis. After adding quality of life factors, although physical abuse severity did not significantly affect resilience, mild physical abuse was more closely associated with resilience as compared to severe physical abuse. These findings are consistent with Dooley et al. (2017), whose previous findings showed a relationship between a moderate level of lifetime stress and resilience, whereas persons with a history of severe distress felt overwhelmed and less resilient. The current study and Dooley et al. (2017) suggest that working through previous hardships (such as mild childhood physical abuse) may better equip the person to successfully work through subsequent difficulties, such as breast cancer.

In terms of the quality-of-life factors, breast cancer survivors in mild and severe physical abuse categories (combined) experienced resilience when they reported current perceived physical limitations, although survivors did not experience resilience when they reported current emotional limitations. Specifically, when survivors experienced emotional limitations, such as believing that mood dysfunction inhibits work productivity and self-care, these survivors were less likely to show resilience. Furthermore, although emotional limitations (in general) negatively impacted resilience, breast cancer survivors who reported worry about recurrence or other breast cancer issues tended to experience resilience. This finding is reasonable and consistent with Fang et al. (2018), who found that fear of recurrence was the most common anxiety in women who had survived cancer for at least 5 years. Therefore, worry about recurrence may potentially be the norm for survivors, including those who are resilient. Emotional limitations as measured by the RAND, however, relate to functional limitations due to depression and anxiety, as opposed to worry about recurrence. This is reasonable to understand in that breast cancer survivors who have difficulty with completing work, chores, and other life activities due to depression and anxiety are less resilient than those who are anxious about recurrence.

Hypothesis 3

The third hypothesis suggested that resilience would be positively associated with posttraumatic growth. Results supported this hypothesis, indicating that resilience was positively associated with posttraumatic growth. Current findings are consistent with Lee et al. (2020), who found a mediating effect between resilience and posttraumatic growth. Specifically, the results of Lee et al. (2020) revealed that the effect of resilience on posttraumatic growth was greatest in the high childhood trauma group, and high levels of resilience were associated with high levels of posttraumatic growth regardless of childhood trauma. Conversely, when resilience was low in the childhood trauma group, posttraumatic growth was low as well. Thus, findings of the current study revealed that breast cancer survivors who showed resilience were also the survivors who achieved posttraumatic growth. This offers a nuanced understanding of the relationship between resilience and posttraumatic growth. Results suggest that the survivors who possess the means to adapt, which is termed resilience, were more likely to achieve a sense of feeling stronger for working through the treatment, which is termed posttraumatic growth. Because resilience is a means of adaptation, which becomes fortified when meeting challenges, the implication is that persons who adjust to strife during childhood, such as abuse, are more likely to grow from struggles in adulthood, such as breast cancer.

Hypothesis 4

Hypothesis 4 suggested that resilience would mediate the association between emotional abuse (in childhood) and posttraumatic growth. In other words, survivors who were emotionally abused were more likely to experience resilience, and resilience of breast cancer survivors who were emotionally abused was associated with significant posttraumatic growth. Although we are well aware of the negative impact of emotional abuse during childhood on psychological wellbeing (Adams et al., 2018), the present study suggests that when persons are able to adapt to emotional adversities that began in childhood, they may become better equipped to grow from traumatic experiences in adulthood, such as breast cancer. Considering this finding, it would be important to examine influences that cause individuals with a history of childhood emotional abuse to develop resilience. With an increased understanding on how resilience can be better fortified in developmental years, mental wellness programs in our educational system can focus upon resilience development.

A Consideration of Specific Findings in the Context of Existing Research

Findings from the current study demonstrated that emotional abuse was significantly and positively associated with posttraumatic growth in breast cancer survivors. Specifically, the greater degree of childhood emotional abuse, the greater degree of posttraumatic growth was seen. Additionally, results indicated that breast cancer survivors who experienced mild and severe childhood physical abuse exhibited more posttraumatic growth than those without physical abuse experiences. The implications of these findings are a departure from the notion that the sole outcome of abusive experiences is psychopathology. While prior research clearly affirms the association between abusive experiences during childhood and psychopathology in adulthood (Adams et al., 2018; Berger et al., 2015; Bretherton, 1992), these current results suggest that in addition to negative outcomes, survivors of childhood abuse may also acquire mental strength and fortitude, which can help them overcome adversities in adulthood. Although the abusive experiences are negative, the ability to withstand adversity can result in the capacity to adapt during adulthood.

Although not included in the hypotheses, a significant finding of the current study was that 87.6% of breast cancer subjects reported a history of childhood physical abuse, with 70.4% in the severe category and 17.2% in the mild category. Only 12.4% of breast cancer subjects did not have a history of childhood abuse. Previous results of the EPAB physical abuse measure revealed severe abuse (33%), mild abuse (54%), and no abuse (12.6%; Wolkins, 2020). Thus, current data are consistent with previous findings that persons with a history of adverse experiences in childhood are at risk for developing cancer. Further, the current study ads specifically recruited breast cancer survivors, versus persons with a history of abusive experiences in childhood. A potential explanation for the higher abuse rate in the current study is that when non-abused survivors initiated the survey, they may have felt uncomfortable with abuse questions. In turn, they have failed to complete the survey, thus increasing/skewing the responses of survivors with an abuse history. Further, breast cancer subjects, who committed to completing the survey, may have been more open and expressive regarding their past, negative experiences as compared to an adult, general population. It would be important to closely examine whether persons with greater degrees of resilience, and posttraumatic growth are more forthcoming regarding past, negative experiences, such as childhood abuse.

Researchers have hypothesized that persons with a history of adverse childhood experiences are prone to chronic stress disorders in their adult lives (Chen & Lacey, 2018). Stress, in turn, activates the sympathetic nervous system, which triggers inflammation, subsequently increasing the risk of developing cancers (Ports et al., 2019). Some persons with a history of childhood maltreatment develop chronic stress-related disorders. Of the individuals who develop chronic stress disorder, some learn to adapt to adverse childhood experiences with resilience. The capacity to determine resilience in response to abusive experiences during childhood has been associated with greater levels of resilience later in life (Fritz et al., 2018). In this regard, breast cancer survivors who have experienced physical abuse are more likely to develop higher posttraumatic growth levels because of their increased resilience and adaptation to traumatic events, such as cancer diagnosis.

The current study found that breast cancer survivors with past physical abuse experiences endorsed multiple individual factors associated with resilience, including cognitive and emotional regulation, social interaction/attachment, and self-concept. The cognitive factors most highly associated with resilience among those breast cancer survivors with high physical abuse experiences compared to those with no physical abuse experience were stronger intellect and cognitive restructuring. Such experiences contribute to improved posttraumatic growth. Emotional regulation, high distress tolerance, low expressive suppression, low aggression, and low alcohol coping expectancy were associated with resilience among breast cancer survivors, resulting in higher posttraumatic growth (Norman et al., 2012). Low insecure attachment, rejection, and other directedness were positively associated with resilience and posttraumatic growth. In the self-concept domain, a balance between low and high ego control and high self-esteem was positively associated with resilience (Fritz et al., 2018). The implication is that past physical abuse experiences among breast cancer survivors provide them with resilience and adaptation to traumatic events, enhancing posttraumatic growth.

When purely examining the association between emotional abuse during childhood and resilience, survivors who were emotionally abused were less likely to experience resilience. Consistent with Dooley et al. (2017), persons with a history of more severe abuse are more likely to feel emotionally overwhelmed, resulting in a negative association with resilience.

When examining the association between emotional abuse during childhood and resilience, while also accounting for survivor's sense of overall wellbeing, survivors with a history of emotional abuse during childhood tended to experience resilience. Specifically, survivors who feel physically and mentally healthy are more likely to experience resilience than those who report that they possess physical and mental limitations. These findings suggest that a survivor's level of resilience may impact perception of physical and mental wellbeing, and also a survivor's sense of physical and mental wellbeing may impact resilience. Thus, in a healthcare environment, screening for breast cancer survivors' perception of their physical and mental health functioning can serve as a reliable predictor for those same survivors' level of resilience.

Current study findings revealed that both mild and severe physical abuse were not associated with resilience. Interestingly, breast cancer survivors with a history of childhood emotional abuse, as opposed to physical abuse, tended to experience resilience. Because resilience is a form of adaptation that becomes further refined when working through challenges, these findings suggest that survivors who are adept at reconciling the harm of emotional abuse are equipped to adapt to the challenges of breast cancer. Thus, from a clinical standpoint, in offering supportive psychotherapy to breast cancer survivors, assessment of the survivor's history of working through negative emotional experiences may help support the patient's adjustment to breast cancer.

The study findings are relevant because they may be useful in determining breast cancer survivors' benefits from psychological care to enhance resilience and promote posttraumatic growth. Further, this study's findings may lead to a greater understanding of how childhood experiences may be harnessed to optimize resilience and posttraumatic growth. Because the severity of adverse experiences during childhood can either thwart or contribute to the associated level of resiliency and posttraumatic growth, it is important to consider the severity of abuse when examining these issues (Hämäläinen & Hari, 2002). Current findings serve as a reminder to clinicians that when offering psychotherapeutic interventions, in addition to assessing current adjustment to breast cancer it is also important to take into consideration the patient's whole life experience extending to adverse experiences during childhood. Thus, results affirm that the events of childhood predict the manner in which we meet the challenges of adulthood. It is important to note that there are numerous psycho-oncology interventions designed to promote PTG in cancer (Eze et al., 2020). Considering the current findings, current programs may be adapted to account for childhood abuse experiences.

The findings are consistent with previous research indicating that it is possible to possess resilience while developing posttraumatic growth (Tedeschi et al., 2018). Resilience is a personal attribute characterized by the ability to bounce back. When described under the lens of posttraumatic growth, resilience refers to the ability of an individual to return to previous levels of functioning (Tedeschi & Blevins, 2015). After experiencing highly stressful, unexpected, negative situations, some individuals grow and transform positively, which refers to posttraumatic growth. While the trauma does not result in posttraumatic growth, posttraumatic growth may occur when persons develop aspects of emotional strength that extend beyond their pre-trauma state (Tedeschi et al., 2018). Positive adaptations can occur following exposure to traumatic events by breast cancer survivors. These positive adaptations include both resilience and posttraumatic growth, where resilience is a coping strategy that helps trauma survivors recover from the aftereffects of stressors (Loeffler et al., 2018). Concurring with the present study's findings, previous literature demonstrates that resilience and posttraumatic growth played a critical and significant role in promoting breast cancer patients' fight for survival, given their ability to withstand harsh treatment (Loeffler et al., 2018).

Concerning resilience and posttraumatic growth, the overall results from the present study indicated that resilience was significantly associated with posttraumatic growth. The findings revealed that resilience was positively associated with posttraumatic growth among breast cancer survivors. The results have also demonstrated that resilience significantly mediates the relationship between emotional abuse and posttraumatic growth among breast cancer survivors. These findings imply that resilience results in higher posttraumatic growth and that experiencing emotional abuse contributes to resilience and increased posttraumatic growth. Prior research also revealed that cancer survivors rated themselves as experiencing greater resilience in social well-being, spirituality, and personal growth than healthy controls (Costanzo et al., 2009). The findings of Costanzo et al. (2009) suggest that cancer survivors endorse resilience in the long term; however, their study did not assess whether adverse experiences before breast cancer contributed to resilience. The findings indicate that persons who can adapt to unfavorable circumstances may help confront future challenges through resilience and higher posttraumatic growth (Dooley et al., 2017).

The current study's findings may be significant for breast cancer survivors, healthcare practitioners, and healthcare facilities in confronting future challenges concerning cancer cases. Current findings are consistent with previous literature, which indicates that persons who can meet struggles with a high degree of resilience can achieve growth because they are mentally stronger for the experience (Li et al., 2020). Li et al. (2020) revealed a significant positive correlation between resilience and posttraumatic growth in breast cancer survivors. In contrast to the current study's results, past research has demonstrated that in addition to posttraumatic growth, resilience showed a significant negative correlation with anxiety and depression and had a positive predictive effect on posttraumatic growth.

Study Limitations

There were several limitations to this study. One of the limitations of the current study is the scoring method for emotional abuse. While physical abuse is classified within one of three finite categories (none, mild, severe), emotional abuse is described by the relationship to the mean. Thus, results can only be described in terms of the degree of the relationship as opposed to finite categories.

The present online study used a self-report survey. Online surveys are the current primary method for collecting data because of this method's ease, the quality of derived data, and access to diverse populations (Jamnik & Lane, 2017). The current study primarily used Facebook for data collection. This platform was selected as Facebook is the largest social network in the United States, and 54% of its users identify as female as of 2022 (Somosi et al., 2023). A specific benefit of data collection via Facebook is the ability to target specific populations (Schneider & Harknett, 2022). With the present study, female breast cancer survivors were specifically targeted. Targeting was utilized because many online breast cancer survivor platforms would not permit administration of the current survey.

There are several limitations to utilizing Facebook for data collection. On the positive side, Facebook use has become ethnically and socio-economically diverse in recent years (Somosi et al., 2023). On the negative side, 86% of Facebook users are between the ages of 18 to 49 (Schneider & Harknett, 2022). Thus, this method of data collection poses limitations in terms of reaching persons in the 50-year-old plus category. It has also been shown that online participants tend to rush in responding to questions, which potentially creates biases in the current dataset (Revilla et al., 2016).

There is an additional relevant note with respect to utilizing a social media platform as a primary means of data collection with this type of survey, wherein subjects are asked to revisit emotional painful experiences. Survivors were presented the option of completing the survey. It would be reasonable to conclude that survivors who are open to emotionally processing negative experiences were inclined to respond, whereas survivors who were less inclined to complete the survey may have not experienced posttraumatic growth. A prior study has shown that subjects are more inclined to respond to social media surveys when they possess a favorable emotional connection with the topic (Ramsey et al., 2016). Therefore, these data may reflect an overrepresentation of resilience and posttraumatic growth in breast cancer survivors.

An additional limitation of the current study is the significant number of respondents who failed to complete the survey. Specifically, more than 40% of participants who started the study did not complete a sufficient number of items, and thus these responses were not included in the analysis. Shorter surveys have been associated with a higher rate of completion (Toepoel & Lugtig, 2022). The important implication regarding the 40% noncompletion rate is that non-abused respondents may have seen the abuse questions as irrelevant, and thus they may have been less motivated in completing the survey. In turn, this may have skewed the data in terms of the notably high abuse rate in the current survey as compared to a general population.

The current survey avoided the use of a specific respondent reward in order to avoid secondary gain as a source of motivation in completing the survey. Although some respondents may be biased in responding based upon financial incentive, the rate of bias tends to be nonsignificant in terms of invalidating responses (Lynch et al, 2019). A limitation of the current study is that survey responses in terms of helping others in need, such as a fellow breast cancer survivor, has not been studied.

Another potential limitation of this study is that, although researcher-defined versus subjective report of childhood abuse is utilized, current responses were based upon retrospective recall of personal, historical events. Previous studies have found that retrospective recall of childhood abuse reported in adulthood was highly associated with psychopathology (Susser & Widom, 2012). Mental health dysfunction was more contingent upon subjective report during adulthood versus medical, legal, and/or psychological official records of abuse; however, because retrospective self-reports are made many years after the maltreatment took place (Widom et al., 2007), bias may occur based upon the impact of early traumatic events on one's ability to recall such events (Newbury et al, 2018). Another significant issue is the potential influence that mood-congruent memory biases could place on the prominence of childhood memories. Thus, respective reporting to determine abusive childhood experiences may not be thoroughly reliable.

Another limitation of the study is that a portion of the findings is based on regression analysis. Because this method was utilized, causal inferences cannot be made. Further, there are likely several other intervening factors associated with resilience and posttraumatic growth that were not examined within the current study. Additionally, this study exclusively examined childhood physical and emotional abuse, while it did not examine other types of adverse experiences such as sexual abuse, neglect, and/or poverty. Future research may wish to include a more comprehensive measurement of childhood experiences that may relate to posttraumatic growth and resiliency.

Applications/Directions for Further Research

Strengthening resilience is an important therapeutic tool (Schulz et al., 2014). This information will be valuable to clinicians in terms of reinforcing the positive. In other words, it may be important for psychologists to help survivors harness and utilize predetermined resilience to help them adjust to the breast cancer experience. Further, these data may also serve as an indicator of persons who may have more difficulty favorably adjusting to the breast cancer experience. For instance, those who perceive with themselves to be less physically and mentally healthy tend to be less resilient and they are less likely to develop posttraumatic growth. These survivors are more likely to require more long-term, intensive treatment from a psychotherapeutic standpoint. Further, as discussed above, the current interventions that emphasize posttraumatic growth in a cancer population may be adapted to account for the impact of the whole life experience, including the effects of childhood experiences.

These findings may also serve as an important reminder that, although there are dire long-term negative outcomes of childhood abuse, individuals who learn to overcome adversity can develop mental fortitude, which may be useful in adapting to difficulties in adulthood. As a clinician, it is important to bear in mind that even when there are long-term negative effects of childhood abuse, these same individuals may also possess strengths that they have acquired from these same adverse experiences. Thus, it is possible for a degree of "damage" and growth to coexist. Additionally, further analysis of the current data set should examine whether there is a curvilinear relationship with emotional abuse because the current analysis is based upon a standard linear regression.

The purpose of the current study was to examine the relationship of abusive experiences during childhood in relation to resilience and posttraumatic growth in breast cancer survivors. Although not contained within the hypothesis, the current survey also examined psychopathology. Future analyses regarding the relationship between resilience, posttraumatic growth, abusive childhood experiences, and psychopathology may be useful. Of particular interest would be to examine the extent to which psychopathology, resilience, and posttraumatic growth can coexist within the current results. Current results cause one to question whether elements of anxiety-related trauma and posttraumatic growth can coexist.

I recommend for further research to be conducted in different geographical regions within the United States to permit the generalizability of findings. Within the current study, 51% of responses were from two states: California (23%) and Pennsylvania (18%). In this regard, future scholars are advised to use inclusive means of analyzing childhood abuse (Carlin et al., 1994; Goldsmith et al., 2009).

The study used a quantitative study design. There are limitations with cross-sectional designs, such as those used in the present study, compared to longitudinal designs. Longitudinal studies are more reliable in addressing both systematic method error due to the use of a single rater or single source and causal inference (Rindfleisch et al., 2008). While a longitudinal study was not possible, a cross-sectional design was appropriate because the study was theoretical, and several measurement instruments were utilized. Further research needs to be conducted using a qualitative design to collect primary data and perceptions of participants regarding their opinions on a given phenomenon. Another limitation of this study was that the study did not investigate whether past stressors can impact posttraumatic growth among people living with breast cancer. The study focused on breast cancer survivors only, excluding other cancer victims or survivors. It is recommended that more studies should be conducted using other cancer survivors or victims to determine the generalizability of this study's findings.

Conclusion

This study aimed to examine the impact of early physical and emotional abuse during childhood on resilience and posttraumatic growth following breast cancer survival. The study demonstrated that breast cancer survivors who had experienced higher emotional abuse exhibited more posttraumatic growth than those without emotional abuse experiences. Both mild abuse and severe physical abuse were also positively associated with posttraumatic growth. Breast cancer survivors who had experienced physical abuse exhibited a higher level of posttraumatic growth than those with no physical abuse. The quality of life, including well-being and breast cancer worry, as well as emotional limitations and perception of general health among breast cancer survivors, were positively associated with resilience.

This study has filled in the gap in the literature by establishing that physical abuse was associated with resilience. Although the findings revealed that mild and severe physical abuse were not associated with resilience, BC QOL Well-Being, BC Worry, RAND Physical Limitations, and Perception of General Health were associated with resilience. Breast cancer survivors with emotional and physical abuse experiences had a high level of resilience, which was significantly associated with posttraumatic growth. Overall, the results demonstrate that resilience significantly mediated the relationship between emotional abuse and posttraumatic growth among breast cancer survivors. I recommend that further research be conducted using a qualitative research design to investigate the relationship between stressors and posttraumatic growth among cancer survivors.

References

Aben, I., Verhey, F., Lousberg, R., Lodder, J., & Honig, A. (2002). Validity of the Beck Depression Inventory, Hospital Anxiety and Depression Scale, SCL-90, and Hamilton Depression Rating Scale as screening instruments for depression in stroke patients. *Psychosomatics*, *43*(5), 386-393.

Adams, J., Mrug, S., & Knight, D. C. (2018). Characteristics of child physical and sexual abuse as predictors of psychopathology. *Child Abuse & Neglect*, *86*, 167–177. https://doi.org/10.1016/j.chiabu.2018.09.019

Allport, G. W. (1961). *Pattern and growth in personality*. Holt, Reinhart & Winston.

American Cancer Society. (2022, March 4). *Breast cancer statistics: How common is breast cancer?* American Cancer Society. Retrieved April 22, 2022, from https://www.cancer.org/cancer/breast-cancer/about/how-common-is-breast-cancer.html#:~:text=Breast%20cancer%20survivors,Survival%20Rates%20for%20Breast%20Cancer

Anders, S. L., Peterson, C. K., James, L. M., Engdahl, B., Leuthold, A. C., & Georgopoulos, A. P. (2015). Neural communication in posttraumatic growth. *Experimental Brain Research*, *233*(7), 2013-2020.

Andrykowski, M. A., Lykins, E., & Floyd, A. (2008, August). Psychological health in cancer survivors. In *Seminars in oncology nursing* (Vol. 24, No. 3, pp. 193-201). WB Saunders.

Asaro, J., Doherty, J., Rehfeld, S., Heimerl, S., Kletkewicz, S., Nagy, J. C., Row, D., Wolkins, R., Carrion, B., Vivian, J., & Fallon, A. (2019, July). *Predicting adult perception of abuse: Examining the sequelae of early abuse and neglect.* [Poster]. Fielding Graduate University, Chicago, Il.

Barber, L. E., Zirpoli, G. R., Cozier, Y. C., Rosenberg, L., Petrick, J. L., Bertrand, K. A., & Palmer, J. R. (2021). Neighborhood disadvantage and individual-level life stressors in relation to breast cancer incidence in US Black women. *Breast Cancer Research, 23*(1), 1-12.

Bellizzi, K. M., & Blank, T. O. (2006). Predicting posttraumatic growth in breast cancer survivors. *Health Psychology*, *25*(1), 47.

Berger, R. P., Parks, S., Fromkin, J., Rubin, P., & Pecora, P. J. (2015). Assessing the accuracy of the International Classification of Diseases codes to identify abusive head trauma: A feasibility study. *Injury Prevention*, *21*(e1), e133-e137.

Blake, D. D., Weathers, F. W., Nagy, L. M., Kaloupek, D. G., Gusman, F. D., Charney, D. S., & Keane, T. M. (1995) The development of a Clinician-Administered PTSD Scale. *Journal of Traumatic Stress*, *8*(1), 75-90. https://doi.org/10.1007/BF02105408

Blevins, C. A., Weathers, F. W., Davis, M. T., Witte, T. K., & Domino, J. L. (2015). The Posttraumatic Stress Disorder Checklist for DSM-5 (PCL-5): Development and initial psychometric evaluation. *Journal of Traumatic Stress, 28*(6). 489-498. https://doi.org/10.1002/jts.22059

Brandão, T., Schulz, M. S., & Matos, P. M. (2017). Psychological adjustment after breast cancer: a systematic review of longitudinal studies. *Psycho-oncology*, *26*(7), 917-926.

Bretherton, I. (1992). The origins of attachment theory: John Bowlby and Mary Ainsworth. *Developmental Psychology*, *28*(5), 759–775. https://doi.org/10.1037/0012-1649.28.5.759

Burnam, M. A., Stein, J. A., Golding, J. M., Siegel, J. M., Sorenson, S. B., Forsythe, A. B., & Telles, C. A. (1988). Sexual assault and mental disorders in a community population. *Journal of Consulting and Clinical Psychology, 56*(6), 843–850. https://doi.org/10.1037/0022-006X.56.6.843

Bush, N. J. (2009). Compassion fatigue: Are you at risk? *Oncology Nursing Forum, 36*(1), 24.

Butler, J., & Kern, M. L. (2016). The PERMA-Profiler: A brief multidimensional measure of flourishing. *International Journal of Wellbeing, 6*(3), 1–48. https://doi.org/10.5502/ijw.v6i3.526

Calhoun, L. G., Cann, A., Tedeschi, R. G., & McMillan, J. (2000). A correlational test of the relationship between posttraumatic growth, religion, and cognitive processing. *Journal of Traumatic Stress: Official Publication of The International Society for Traumatic Stress Studies, 13*(3), 521-527.

Cann, A., Calhoun, L. G., Tedeschi, R. G., & Solomon, D. T. (2010). Posttraumatic growth and depreciation as independent experiences and predictors of well-being. *Journal of Loss and Trauma, 15(3),* 151-166.

Carlin, A. S., Kemper, K., Ward, N. G., Sowell, H., Gustafson, B., & Stevens, N. (1994). The effect of differences in objective and subjective definitions of childhood physical abuse on estimates of its incidence and relationship to psychopathology. *Child Abuse & Neglect, 18*(5), 393-399.

Carr, A., Duff, H., & Craddock, F. (2020). A systematic review of reviews of the outcome of noninstitutional child maltreatment. *Trauma, Violence, & Abuse*, *21*(4), 828-84.

Chan, P. F., & Abd Hamid, R. (2021). An overview of breast cancer: Classification and related signaling pathways. *Progress In Microbes & Molecular Biology*, *4*(1), 14-22.

Chen, M., & Lacey, R. E. (2018). Adverse childhood experiences and adult inflammation: Findings from the 1958 British birth cohort. *Brain, Behavior, and Immunity*, *69*, 582-590. https://doi.org/10.1016/j.bbi.2018.02.007

Child Welfare Information Gateway. (2019). *Definitions of child abuse and neglect.* U.S. Department of Health and Human Services, Children's Bureau.

Child Welfare Information Gateway. (2014). *Definitions of child abuse and neglect.* U.S. Department of Health and Human Services, Children's Bureau.

Clarke, P. J., Notebaert, L., & MacLeod, C. (2014). Absence of evidence or evidence of absence: reflecting on therapeutic implementations of attentional bias modification. *BMC psychiatry*, *14*, 1-6.

Connor, K. M., & Davidson, J. R. (2003). Development of a new resilience scale: The Connor-Davidson Resilience Scale (CD-RISC). *Depression and Anxiety, 18*(2), 76-82. https://doi.org/10.1002/da.10113

Costanzo, E. S., Ryff, C. D., & Singer, B. H. (2009). Psychosocial adjustment among cancer survivors: Findings from a national survey of health and well-being. *Health Psychology*, *28*(2), 147-164.

Davidson, R. J., & Begley, S. (2012). *The emotional life of your brain: How its unique patterns affect the way you think, feel, and live, and how you can change them.* Hudson Street Press.

Derogatis, L. R. (1983). *SCL-90-R administration, scoring & procedures manual-II.* Clinical Psychometric Research.

Derogatis, L. R. (2000). *Symptom Checklist-90-Revised. Handbook of psychiatric measures.* American Psychiatric Association.

Derogatis L. R., Rickles K., & Rock A. F. (1976). The SCL-90 and the MMPI: A step in the validation of a new self-report study. *British Journal of Psychiatry, 128*, 280-289.

Derogatis L. R. & Savitz K. L. (1999). The SCL-90-R, Brief Symptom Inventory and matching clinical rating scales. In M.E. Maruish, *The use of psychological testing for treatment planning and outcomes assessment*, pp. 679-724, Lawrence Erlbaum.

Di Giacomo, D., Cannita, K., Ranieri, J., Cocciolone, V., Passafiume, D., & Ficorella, C. (2016). Breast cancer and psychological resilience among young women. *Journal of Psychopathology, 3*(1), 9001-9005.

Dockray, S., & Steptoe, A. (2010). Positive affect and psychobiological processes. *Neuroscience and Biobehavioral Reviews, 35*(1), 69–75.

Doherty, J., Dwyer, B., Kletkewicz, S., Lapinski, K., Dao, L., Wolkins, R., & Fallon, A. (2022, January). *Perception of adverse experiences throughout the lifespan and its impact on interpersonal sensitivity in adulthood.* [Poster]. Fielding Graduate University. Santa Barbara, California.

Dooley, L. N., Slavich, G. M., Moreno, P. I., & Bower, J. E. (2017). Strength through adversity: Moderate lifetime stress exposure is associated with psychological resilience in breast cancer survivors. *Stress and Health, 33*(5), 549-557.

Drageset, S., Lindstrøm, T. C., & Underlid, K. (2010). Coping with breast cancer: Between diagnosis and surgery. *Journal of Advanced Nursing, 66*(1), 149-158.

Etikan, I., Musa, S. A., & Alkassim, R. S. (2016). Comparison of convenience sampling and purposive sampling. *American Journal of Theoretical and Applied Statistics, 5*(1), 1-4.

Eze, J. E., Ifeagwazi, C. M., & Chukwuorji, J. C. (2020). Core beliefs challenge and posttraumatic growth: Mediating role of rumination among internally displaced survivors of terror attacks. *Journal of Happiness Studies*, *21*, 659-676.

Fang, S. Y., Fetzer, S. J., Lee, K.T., & Kuo, Y. L. (2018). Fear of recurrence as a predictor of care needs for long-term breast cancer survivors. *Cancer Nursing*, *41*(1), 69-76.

Felitti, V. J., Anda, R. F., Nordenberg, D., Spitz, A. M., Edwards, V., Koss, M. P., & Marks, J.S. (1998). Relationship of childhood abuse and household dysfunction to many of the leading causes of death in adults. The Adverse Childhood Experiences (ACE) Study. *American Journal of Preventative Medicine, 14*(4), 245-258. https://doi.org/10.1016/s0749-3797(98)00017-8

First, M. B., Spitzer, R. L., Gibbon, M., & Williams, J. B. W. (2002). Structured clinical interview for DSM-IV-TR Axis I disorders, research version, patient edition (SCID-I/P). *Biometrics Research.*

Fitch, M. I., Osoba, D., Iscoe, N., & Szalai, J. P. (1995). Predicting psychological distress in patients with cancer: Conceptual basis and reliability evaluation of a self-report questionnaire. *Anticancer Research, 15*(4), 1533-1542.

Frankl, V. E. (1985). *Man's search for meaning*. Simon and Schuster.

Fritz, J., De Graaff, A. M., Caisley, H., Van Harmelen, A. L., & Wilkinson, P. O. (2018). A systematic review of amenable resilience factors that moderate and/or mediate the relationship between childhood adversity and mental health in young people. *Frontiers in Psychiatry*, *9*, 230-252.

Fritz, M. S., & MacKinnon, D. P. (2007). Required sample size to detect the mediated effect. *Psychological Science*, *18*(3), 233-239.

Galinowski A., Miranda R., Lemaitre H., Paillère Martinot M. L., Artiges E., Vulser H., Goodman R., Penttilä J., Struve M., Barbot A., Fadai T., Poustka L., Conrod P., Banaschewski T., Barker G. J., Bokde A., Bromberg U., Büchel C., Flor H.,...Martinot J. L. (2015). Resilience and corpus collosum microstructure in adolescence. *Psychological Medicine, 45*(11), 2285-2294. https://doi.org/10.1017/S0033291715000239

Gangstad, B., Norman, P., & Barton, J. (2009). Cognitive processing and posttraumatic growth after stroke. *Rehabilitation Psychology, 54*(1), 69-82.

Gathani, T., Clayton, G., MacInnes, E., & Horgan, K. (2021). The COVID-19 pandemic and impact on breast cancer diagnoses: What happened in England in the first half of 2020. *British Journal of Cancer, 124*(4), 710-712.

Giuliano, A. E., Edge, S. B., & Hortobagyi, G. N. (2018). Eighth edition of the AJCC Cancer Staging Manual: Breast Cancer. *Annals of Surgical Oncology, 25*(7), 1783-1785.

Greene, F. L., & Kosinski, L. A. (2018). Cancer staging. *The American Cancer Society's Principles of Oncology: Prevention to Survivorship, 35*(5), 184-190.

Goldsmith, R. E., Freyd, J. J., & DePrince, A. P. (2009). To add insight to injury: Childhood abuse, abuse perceptions, and the emotional and physical health of young adults. *Journal of Aggression, Maltreatment & Trauma, 18*(4), *350-366.*

Grogan, S., & Mechan, J. (2017). Body image after mastectomy: A thematic analysis of younger women's written accounts. *Journal of Health Psychology, 22*(11), 1480-1490.

Guil, R., Ruiz-González, P., Merchán-Clavellino, A., Morales-Sánchez, L., Zayas, A., & Gómez-Molinero, R. (2020). Breast cancer and resilience: The controversial role of perceived emotional intelligence. *Frontiers in Psychology, 11*, 595713.

Gupta, A., Love, A., Kilpatrick, L. A., Labus, J. S., Bhatt, R., Chang, L., Tillisch, K., Naliboff, B., & Mayer, E. A. (2017). Morphological brain measures of cortico-limbic inhibition related to resilience. *Journal of Neuroscience Research, 95*(9), 1760–1775.

Hafkenscheid, A. (1993). Psychometric evaluation of the Symptom Checklist (SCL-90) in psychiatric patients. *Personality and Individual Differences, 14*(6), 751–756. https://doi.org/10.1016/0191-8869(93)90088-K

Hämäläinen, M., & Hari, R. (2002). Magnetoencephalographic characterization of dynamic brain activation: Basic principles and methods of data collection and source analysis. In *Brain Mapping: The Methods* (2nd ed., pp. 227-253). Elsevier Science Inc.

Hayes, A. F. (2018). *Introduction to mediation, moderation, and conditional process analysis: A regression-based approach (methodology in the social sciences)* (2nd ed.). The Guilford Press.

Higgins, D. J., & McCabe, M. P. (2001). Multiple forms of child abuse and neglect: Adult retrospective reports. *Aggression and Violent Behavior, 6*(6), 547–578. https://doi.org/10.1016/S1359-1789(00)00030-6.

Hill, E. M., & Watkins, K. (2017). Women with ovarian cancer: Examining the role of social support and rumination in posttraumatic growth, psychological distress, and psychological well-being. *Journal of Clinical Psychology in Medical Settings, 24*(1), 47-58.

Horowitz, M., Wilner, N., & Alvarez, W. (1979) Impact of Event Scale: A measure of subjective stress. *Psychosomatic Medicine, 41*(3), 209-218. https://doi.org/10.1097/00006842-197905000-00004

Hovdestad, W. E., Shields, M., Shaw, A., & Tonmyr, L. (2020). Childhood maltreatment as a risk factor for cancer: Findings from a population-based survey of Canadian adults. *BMC Cancer*, *20*(1), 70-84.

Hunter, R. G., Gray, J. D., & McEwen, B. S. (2018). The neuroscience of resilience. *Journal of the Society for Social Work and Research*, *9*(2), 305-339.

Infurna, F. J., & Jayawickreme, E. (2019). Fixing the growth illusion: New directions for research in resilience and posttraumatic growth. *Current Directions in Psychological Science*, *28*(2), 152–158. https://doi.org/10.1177/0963721419827017

Islami, F., Guerra, C. E., Minihan, A., Yabroff, K. R., Fedewa, S. A., Sloan, K., Wiedt, T. L., Thomson, B., Siegel, R. L., Nargis, N., Winn, R. A., Lacasse, L., Makeroff, L., Daniels, E. C., Patel, A. V., Cance, W. G., & Jemal, A. (2022). American Cancer Society's report on the status of cancer disparities in the United States, 2021. *CA: A Cancer Journal for Clinicians*, *72*(2), 112-143.

Jamnik, M. R., & Lane, D. J. (2017). The use of Reddit as an inexpensive source for high-quality data. *Practical Assessment, Research, & Evaluation, 22*(1). https://doi.org/10.7275/j18t-c009

Jankovic, C., Sharp, J., & Thielking, M. (2022). Child maltreatment and post-traumatic growth: Implications for the well-being of young adults. *Child Abuse & Neglect*, *131*, 105783.

Jayawickreme, E., Infurna, F. J., Alajak, K., Blackie, L. E., Chopik, W. J., Chung, J. M., Dorfman, A., Fleeson, W., Forgeard, M. J., Frazier, P., Furr, R. M., Grossmann, I., Heller, A. S., Laceulle, O. M., Lucas, R. E., Luhmann, M., Luong, G., Meijer, L., McLean, K. C., … Zonneveld, R. (2020). Post-traumatic growth as positive personality change: Challenges, opportunities, and recommendations. *Journal of Personality*, *89*(1), 145–165. https://doi.org/10.1111/jopy.12591

Jones, G. (2002). What is this thing called mental toughness? An investigation of elite sport performers. *Journal of Applied Sport Psychology*, *14*(3), 205-218.

Kangas M. (2013). DSM-5 trauma and stress-related disorders: Implications for screening for cancer-related stress. *Frontiers in Psychiatry*, *4*, 122-126.

Kessler, R. C., Stang, P. E., Wittchen, H. U., Ustun T. B., Roy-Burne, P. P., & Walters, E. E. (1998) Lifetime panic-depression comorbidity in the National Comorbidity Survey. *Archives of General Psychiatry, 55*(9), 801-808. https://doi.org/10.1001/archpsyc.55.9.801

Keyes, C. L. M. (1998). Social well-being. *Social Psychology Quarterly, 61*(2), 121-140. https://doi.org/10.2307/2787065

Khoshouei, M. S. (2009). Psychometric evaluation of the Connor-Davidson Resilience Scale (CD-RISC) using Iranian students. *International Journal of Testing*, *9*(1), 60-66.

Kiełb, K., Bargiel-Matusiewicz, K. M., & Pisula, E. (2019). Posttraumatic stress symptoms and posttraumatic growth in mothers of children with intellectual disability – The role of intrusive and deliberate ruminations: A preliminary report. *Frontiers in Psychology*, *10*. https://doi.org/10.3389/fpsyg.2019.02011

Klassen, A. F., Kaur, M. N., Tsangaris, E., de Vries, C. E., Bordeleau, L., Zhong, T., Cano, S. J., Breitkopfm T., & Pusic, A. L. (2021). Development and psychometric validation of BREAST-Q Scales measuring cancer worry, fatigue, and impact on work. *Annals of Surgical Oncology*, *28*(12), 7410-7420.

Knutson, J. F., & Selner, M. B. (1994). Punitive childhood experiences reported by young adults over a 10-year period. *Child Abuse & Neglect, 18*(2), 155–166. https://doi.org/10.1016/0145- 2134(94)90117-1

Kuldas, S., & Foody, M. (2022). Neither resiliency-trait nor resilience-state: Transactional Resiliency/e. *Youth & Society*, *54*(8), 1352-1376.

Lazaraton, A. (2005). Quantitative research methods. In E. Hinkel (Ed.) *Handbook of research in second language teaching and learning* (pp. 233-248). Routledge.

Lee, D., Yu, E. S., & Kim, N. H. (2020). Resilience as a mediator in the relationship between posttraumatic stress and posttraumatic growth among adult accident or crime victims: The moderated mediating effect of childhood trauma. *European Journal of Psychotraumatology*, *11*(1), 1704563.

Leung, J., McKenzie, S., Martin, J., & McLaughlin, D. (2014). Effect of rurality on screening for breast cancer: A systematic review and meta-analysis comparing mammography. *Rural and Remote Health*, *14*(2), 260-272.

Li, L., Hou, Y., Kang, F., & Wei, X. (2020). The mediating and moderating roles of resilience in the relationship between anxiety, depression, and posttraumatic growth among breast cancer patients based on structural equation modeling: An observational study. *Medicine*, *99*(50), e23273.

Linde-Krieger, L. B., Moon, C. M., & Yates, T. M. (2021). The implications of self-definitions of child sexual abuse for understanding socioemotional adaptation in young adulthood. *Journal of Child Sexual Abuse*, *30*(1), 80-101.

Locke, H. J., & Wallace, K. M. (1959). Short marital-adjustment and prediction tests: Their reliability and validity. *Marriage & Family Living, 21*, 251–255. https://doi.org/10.2307/348022

Loeffler, S., Poehlmann, K., & Hornemann, B. (2018). Finding meaning in suffering? Meaning making and psychological adjustment over the course of a breast cancer disease. *European Journal of Cancer Care*, *27*(3), e12841.

Lynch, H. F., Joffe, S., Thirumurthy, H., Xie, D., & Largent, E. A. (2019). Association between financial incentives and participant deception about study eligibility. *Jama Network Open* *2*(1), https://doi.org/10.1001/jamanetworkopen.2018.7355

Maitlis, S. (2020). Posttraumatic growth at work. *Annual Review of Organizational Psychology and Organizational Behavior*, *7*(1), 395–419. https://doi.org/10.1146/annurev-orgpsych-012119-044932

Mandelli, L., Petrelli, C., & Serretti, A. (2015). The role of specific early trauma in adult depression: A meta-analysis of published literature. Childhood trauma and adult depression. *European Psychiatry*, *30*(6), 665-680.

Marks, D. F., Murray, M., & Vida Estacio, E. (2015). *Health psychology: Theory, research, & practice,* (5th ed). Sage Publications. ISBN 978-1-5264-0823-5 ISBN 978-1-5264-0824-2 (pbk)

Martínez-Martí, M. L., & Ruch, W. (2017). Character strengths predict resilience over and above positive affect, self-efficacy, optimism, social support, self-esteem, and life satisfaction. *The Journal of Positive Psychology, 12*(2), 110-119.

Masten, A., Motti-Stefanidi, F., & Rahl-Brigman, H. (2019). Developmental risk and resilience in the context of devastation and forced migration. In R. Parke & G. Elder, Jr. (Eds.), *Children in changing worlds: Sociocultural and temporal perspectives* (pp. 84-111). Cambridge University Press. https://doi.org/:10.1017/9781108264846.004

McDonough, M. H., Sabiston, C. M., & Wrosch, C. (2014). Predicting changes in posttraumatic growth and subjective well-being among breast cancer survivors: The role of social support and stress. *Psycho-Oncology, 23*(1), 114-120.

Meston, C. M., Heiman, J. R., Trapnell, P. D., & Carlin, A. S. (1999). Ethnicity, desirable responding, and self-reports of abuse: a comparison of European-and Asian-ancestry undergraduates. *Journal of Consulting and Clinical Psychology, 67*(1), 139.

Millon, T., Krueger, R. F., & Simonsen, E. (2010). *Contemporary directions in psychopathology: Scientific foundations of the DSM-5 and ICD-11*. Guilford.

Mohr, D., & Rosén, L. A. (2017). The impact of protective factors on posttraumatic growth for college student survivors of childhood maltreatment. *Journal of Aggression, Maltreatment & Trauma, 26*(7), 756-771.

Momenimovahed, Z., & Salehiniya, H. (2019). Epidemiological characteristics of and risk factors for breast cancer in the world. *Breast Cancer (Dove Medical Press), 11*, 151–164. https://doi.org/10.2147/BCTT.S176070

Muela, A., Barandiaran, A., de Arana, E. L., Larrea, I., & Vitoria, J. R. (2012). *Definition, incidence and psychopathological consequences of child abuse and neglect*. INTECH Open Access Publisher.

Nagy, C., Kletkewicz, S., Heimerl, S., Rehfeld, S.M., Row, D., Wolkins, R., Aaron, J., Asaro, J., Carrion, B., Cornelius, C., & Fallon, A. (2019). *It's my normal: Does socioeconomic status moderate the relationship between perceived abuse and actual abuse?* (poster) Fielding Graduate University, Santa Barbara, CA.

Newbury, J. B., Arseneault, L., Moffitt, T. E., Caspi, A., Danese, A., Baldwin, J. R., & Fisher, H. L. (2018). Measuring childhood maltreatment to predict early-adult psychopathology: Comparison of prospective informant-reports and retrospective self-reports. *Journal of Psychiatric Research, 96*, 57-64.

Niakan, S., Love, H., Lipoff, D., Casaubon, J., & Mason, H. (2021). Best practices in breast health and breast cancer screening. *Advances in Family Practice Nursing, 3*, 121-133. Oncology Nursing Society.

Norman, R. E., Byambaa, M., De, R., Butchart, A., Scott, J., & Vos, T. (2012). The long-term health consequences of child physical abuse, emotional abuse, and neglect: A systematic review and meta-analysis. *PLoS Medicine*, *9*(11), e1001349.

Oettingen, G., & Wadden, T. A. (1991). Expectation, fantasy, and weight loss: Is the impact of positive thinking always positive? *Cognitive Therapy and Research, 15*(2), 167–175. https://doi.org/10.1007/BF01173206

Ogińska-Bulik, N., & Kobylarczyk, M. (2017). The mediating role of resiliency in the relationship between temperament and posttraumatic growth. *Journal of Loss and Trauma*, *22*(1), 1-10.

Ports, K. A., Holman, D. M., Guinn, A. S., Pampati, S., Dyer, K. E., Merrick, M. T., Lunsford, N. B., & Metzler, M. (2019). Adverse childhood experiences and the presence of cancer risk factors in adulthood: A scoping review of the literature from 2005 to 2015. *Journal of Pediatric Nursing, 44*, 81–96. https://doi.org/10.1016/j.pedn.2018.10.009

Preston A. R., & Eichenbaum, H. (2013) Interplay of hippocampus and prefrontal cortex in memory. *Current Biology, 23*(17), R764-73. https://doi.org/10.1016/j.cub.2013.05.041.

Puetz, V. B., Viding, E., Maguire, E. A:, Mechelli, A., Armbruster-Genç, D., Sharp, M., Rankin, G., Gerin, M. I., & McCrory, E. J. (2021). Functional brain plasticity following childhood maltreatment: A longitudinal fMRI investigation of autobiographical memory processing. *Development and Psychopathology, 35*(3), 1-8.

Pusic, A. L., Klassen, A. F., Scott, A. M., Klok, J. A., Cordeiro, P. G., & Cano, S. J. (2009). Development of a new patient-reported outcome measure for breast surgery: The BREAST-Q. *Plastic and Reconstructuctive Surgery, 124*(2), 345-353. https://doi.org/10.1097/PRS.0b013e3181aee807

Quintana, C. (2014). *Perceptions and experiences of physical punishment in childhood and their subsequent impact on social and psychological functioning in American and Mexican populations* (Order No. 3623651). Available from Dissertations & Theses @ Fielding Graduate University.

Ramsey, S. R., Thompson, K. L., McKenzie, M., & Rosenbaum, A. (2016). Psychological research in the internet age: The quality of web-based data. *Computers in Human Behavior, 58*, 354-360.

Rausch, K., & Knutson, J. F. (1991). The self-report of personal punitive childhood experiences and those of siblings. *Child Abuse & Neglect, 15*(1/2), 29–36. https://doi.org/10.1016/0145- 2134(91)90087-

Rauter, U. K., Leonard, C. E., & Swett, C. P. (1995). SCL-90-R factor structure in an acute, involuntary, adult psychiatric inpatient samples. *Journal of Clinical Psychology, 52*(6), 625-629. https://doi.org/10.1002/(sici)1097-4679(199611)52:6%3C625::aid-jclp4%3E3.0.co;2-j

Reuben, A., Moffitt, T. E., Caspi, A., Belsky, D. W., Harrington, H., Schroeder, F., Hogan, S., Ramrakha, S., Poulton, R., & Danese, A. (2016). Lest we forget: Comparing retrospective and prospective assessments of adverse childhood experiences in the prediction of adult health. *Journal of Child Psychology and Psychiatry, and Allied Disciplines, 57(*10), 1103-12. https://doi.org/10.1111/jcpp.12621.

Revilla, M., Toninelli, D., Ochoa, C., & Loewe, G. (2016). Do online access panels need to adapt surverys for mobile devices? *Internet Research, 26*(5), 1209-1227.

Rindfleisch, A., Malter, A. J., Ganesan, S., & Moorman, C. (2008). Cross-sectional versus longitudinal survey research: Concepts, findings, and guidelines. *Journal of Marketing Research, 45*(3), 261-279.

Rogers, C. R. (1951). *Client-centered therapy; its current practice, implications, and theory.* Houghton Mifflin.

Rossouw, J. G., Rossouw, P. J., Paynter, C., Ward, A., & Khnana, P. (2017). Predictive 6 factor resilience scale-Domains of resilience and their role as enablers of job satisfaction. *International Journal of Neuropsychotherapy, 2*(1), 25-40.

Rossouw, P. J., & Rossouw, J. G. (2016). The predictive 6-factor resilience scale: Neurobiological fundamentals and organizational application. *International Journal of Neuropsychotherapy*, *4*(1), 31-45.

Rowland, J. H. (2007). Survivorship research: Past, present, and future. In P.A. Ganz (Ed.), *Cancer survivorship* (pp. 28-42). Springer.

Rozentsvit, I. (2016). The post-traumatic growth: The wisdom of the mind, its clinical and neuropsychoanalytic vicissitudes. *European Psychiatry, 33*(S1), S568-S568. https://doi.org/10.1016/j.eurpsy.2016.01.2105

Ryff, C. D., & Keyes, C. L. M. (1995). The structure of psychological well-being revisited. *Journal of Personality and Social Psychology*, *69*(4), 719-734.

Rytilä-Manninen, M., Fröjd, S., Haravuori, H., Lindberg, N., Marttunen, M., Kettunen, K., & Therman S. (2016). Psychometric properties of the Symptom Checklist-90 in adolescent psychiatric inpatients and age- and gender-matched community youth. *Childhood and Psychiatry and Mental Health. 10*(3), 121-133.

Salovey, P., Mayer, J. D., Goldman, S. L., Turvey, C., & Palfai, T. P. (1995). Emotional attention, clarity, and repair: Exploring emotional intelligence using the Trait Meta-Mood Scale. In J. W. Pennebaker (Ed.), *Emotion, disclosure, & health* (pp. 125–154). American Psychological Association. https://doi.org/10.1037/10182-006

Schaefer, L. M., Howell, K. H., Schwartz, L. E., Bottomley, J. S., & Crossnine, C. B. (2018). A concurrent examination of protective factors associated with resilience and posttraumatic growth following childhood victimization. *Child Abuse & Neglect*, *85*, 17-27.

Schlatter, M. C., & Cameron, L. D. (2010). Emotional suppression tendencies as predictors of symptoms, mood, and coping appraisals during AC chemotherapy for breast cancer treatment. *Annals of Behavioral Medicine*, *40*(1), 15-29.

Schneider, D., & Harknett, K. (2022). What's to like? Facebook as a tool for survey data collection. *Sociological Methods & Research*, *51*(1), 108-140.

Schore, A. N. (2000). Attachment and the regulation of the right brain. *Attachment & Human Development, 2,* 23–47.

Schulz, A., Becker, M., Van der Auwera, S., Barnow, S., Appel, K., Mahler, J., Schmidt, C. O., Ulrich, J., Freyberger, H. J., & Grabe, H. J. (2014). The impact of childhood trauma on depression: Does resilience matter?: Population-based results from the Study of Health in Pomerania. *Journal of Psychosomatic Research*, *77*(2), 97-103.

Seery, M. D., Holman, E. A., & Silver, R. C. (2010). Whatever does not kill us: Cumulative lifetime adversity, vulnerability, and resilience. *Journal of Personality & Social Psychology, 99*(6), 1025-1041. https://doi.org/10.1037/a0021344

Sharma, S., Wong, D., Schomberg, J., Knudsen-Robbins, C., Gibbs, D., Berkowitz, C., & Heyming, T. (2021). COVID-19: Differences in sentinel injury and child abuse reporting during a pandemic. *Child Abuse & Neglect*, *26*(11), 116-127.

Shonkoff, J. P. (2016). Capitalizing on advances in science to reduce the health consequences of early childhood adversity. *JAMA Pediatrics*, *170*(10), 1003-1007. https://jamanetwork.com/journals/jamapediatrics/article-abstract/2546141

Silvern, L., Waelde, L. C., Baughan, B. M., Karyl, J., & Kaersvang, L. L. (2000). Two formats for eliciting retrospective reports of child sexual and physical abuse: Effects on apparent prevalence and relationships to adjustment. *Child Maltreatment, 5*(3), 236-250. https://doi.org/10.1177/1077559500005003004

Simeon, D., Yehuda, R., Cunill, R., Knutelska, M., Putnam, F. W., & Smith, L. M. (2007). Factors associated with resilience in healthy adults. *Psychoneuroendocrinology*, *32*(8-10), 1149-1152.

Silva, S. M., Moreira, H. C., & Canavarro, M. C. (2012). Examining the links between perceived impact of breast cancer and psychosocial adjustment: The buffering role of posttraumatic growth. *Psycho-Oncology*, *21*(4), 409-418.

Slade, M., Rennick-Egglestone, S., Blackie, L., Llewellyn-Beardsley, J., Franklin, D., Hui, A., Thornicroft, G., McGranahan, R., Pollock, K., Priebe, S., Ramsay, A., Roe, D., & Deakin, E. (2019). Posttraumatic growth in mental health recovery: Qualitative study of narratives. *BMJ Open*, *9*(6). 27-42. https://doi.org/10.1136/bmjopen-2019-029342

Slavich, G. M., & Toussaint, L. (2014). Using the Stress and Adversity Inventory as a teaching tool leads to significant learning gains in two courses on stress and health. *Stress & Health 30*(4), 343–352. https://doi.org/10.1002/smi.2523

Somosi, Z., Hajdú, N., & Molnár, L. (2023). Targeting in online marketing: A retrospective analysis with a focus on practices of Facebook, Google, LinkedIn and TikTok. *European Journal of Business and Management Research*, *8*(1), 33-39.

Spiegel, D. (2012). Mind matters in cancer survival. *Psycho-Oncology*, *21*(6), 588-593.

Stanton, A. L., Revenson, T. A., & Tennen, H. (2007). Health psychology: Psychological adjustment to chronic disease. *Annual Reviews of Psychology*, *58*, 565-592.

Stava, C., Weiss, L. T., & Vassilopoulou-Sellin, R. (2006). Health profiles of 814 very long-term breast cancer survivors. *Clinical Breast Cancer, 7*(3), 228-236.

Stump-Sutliff, K. A. (2022, March 2). *Breast cancer: What are the survival rates?* WebMD. Retrieved April 22, 2022, from https://www.webmd.com/breast-cancer/guide/breast-cancersurvivalrates#:~:text=The%20overall%205%2Dyear%20relative,are%20alive%20after%2010%20years).

Susser, E., & Widom, C. S. (2012). Still searching for lost truths about the bitter sorrows of childhood. *Schizophrenia Bulletin, 38*(4), 672-675.

Swainston, J., Chapman, B., Grunfeld, E. A., & Derakshan, N. (2020). COVID-19 lockdown and its adverse impact on psychological health in breast cancer. *Frontiers in Psychology, 11*, 2033.

Taku, K., Cann, A., Calhoun, L. G., & Tedeschi, R. G. (2008). The factor structure of the Posttraumatic Growth Inventory: A comparison of five models using confirmatory factor analysis. *Journal of Traumatic Stress, 21*(2), 158-164.

Taylor, S.E., Lichtman, R. R., Wood, J. V. (1984). Attributions, beliefs about control, and adjustment to breast cancer. *Journal of Personality and Social Psychology, 46*(3), 489-502. https://doi.org/10.1037//0022-3514.46.3.489

Tedeschi, R. G., & Blevins, C. L. (2015). From mindfulness to meaning: Implications for the theory of posttraumatic growth. *Psychological Inquiry, 26*(4), 373-376.

Tedeschi, R. G., Blevins, C. L., & Riffle, O. M. (2017). Posttraumatic growth: A brief history and evaluation. In M. A. Warren & S. I. Donaldson (Eds.), *Scientific advances in positive psychology* (pp. 131–163). Praeger/ABC-CLIO.

Tedeschi, R. G., & Calhoun, L. G. (1995). *Trauma and transformation.* Sage Publications.

Tedeschi, R. G., & Calhoun, L. G. (1996). The Posttraumatic Growth Inventory: Measuring the positive legacy of trauma. *Journal of Traumatic Stress*, *9*(3), 455-471.

Tedeschi, R. G., & Calhoun, L. G. (2004). Posttraumatic growth: Conceptual foundations and empirical evidence. *Psychological Inquiry*, *15*(1), 1-18.

Tedeschi, R. G., Shakespeare-Finch, J., Taku, K., & Calhoun, L. G. (2018). *Posttraumatic growth: Theory, research and applications*. Routledge.

Teicher, M. H., & Samson, J. A. (2016). Annual research review: Enduring neurobiological effects of childhood abuse and neglect. *Journal of Child Psychology and Psychiatry*, *57*(3), 241-266.

Toepoel, V., & Lugtig, P. (2022). Modularization in an era of mobile web: Investigating the effects of cutting a survey into smaller pieces on data quality. *Social Science Computer Review, 40*(1), 150-164. https://doi.org/10.1177/0894439318784882

Tranter, H., Brooks, M., & Khan, R. (2020). Emotional resilience and event centrality mediate posttraumatic growth following adverse childhood experiences. *Psychological Trauma: Theory, Research, Practice, and Policy*, *13*(2), 165–173.

Trayes, K. P., & Cokenakes, S. E. (2021). Breast cancer treatment. *American Family Physician*, *104*(2), 171-178.

The United States Children's Bureau. (2022) *Child Welfare Survey.* United States Department of Health and Human Services. https://www.childstats.gov/americaschildren/index8.asp

Velentgas, P., Dreyer, N. A., & Wu, A.W. (2013). Outcome definition and measurement. In P. Velentgas, N. A. Dreyer, P., Nourjah, S. R., Smith, & M. M. Torchia (Eds.). *Developing a protocol for observational comparative effectiveness research: A user's guide.* Agency for Healthcare Research and Quality. http://www.ncbi.nlm.nih.gov/books/NBK126186

Wagnild, G. M., & Young, H. M. (1993). Development and psychometric evaluation of the Resilience Scale. *Journal of Nursing Measurement, 1*(2), 165–178.

Waks, A. G., & Winer, E. P. (2019). Breast cancer treatment: A review. *Journal of the American Medical Association, 321*(3), 288-300.

Ware J. E., & Sherbourne, C. D. (1992). The MOS 36-item short-form health survey (SF-36). I. Conceptual framework and item selection. *Medical Care, 30*(6), 473-483.

Watson, D., Clark, L. A., & Tellegen, A. (1988). Development and validation of brief measures of positive and negative affect: the PANAS scales. *Journal of Personality and Social Psychology, 54*(6):1063-1070. https://doi.org/10.1037//0022-3514.54.6.1063

Widom, C.S., DuMont, K., & Czaja, S. J. (2007). A prospective investigation of major depressive disorder and comorbidity in abused and neglected children grown up. *Archives of General Psychiatry, 64*(1), 49-56. https://doi.org/10.1001/archpsyc.64.1.49

Wolkins, R. D. (2020). *The operationalization and measurement of childhood physical abuse: An examination of the relationship of researcher and subjective definitions of childhood physical abuse and adult psychopathology* [Doctoral , Fielding Graduate University].

Wu X., Kaminga, A. C., Dai, W., Deng, J., Wang, Z., Pan, X., & Liu, A. (2019). The prevalence of moderate-to-high posttraumatic growth: A systematic review and meta-analysis. *Journal of Affective Disorders, 243*, 408-415. https://doi.org/10.1016/j.jad.2018.09.023

Yu, X.N., & Zhang, J.X. (2007) A comparison between the Chinese version of Ego-Resiliency Scale and Connor-Davidson Resilience Scale. *Psychological Science (China), 30*(5), 1169-1171.

Zack, M., Toneatto, T., & Streiner, D. L. (1998). The SCL-90 factor structure in comorbid substance abusers. *Journal of Substance Abuse, 10*(1), 85–101. https://doi.org/10.1016/S0899-3289(99)80143-6

Zebrack, B., Kwak, M., Salsman, J., Cousino, M., Meeske, K., Aguilar, C., Embry, L, Block, R., Hayes-Lattin, B., & Cole, S. (2015). The relationship between posttraumatic stress and posttraumatic growth among adolescent and young adult (AYA) cancer patients. *Psycho-Oncology*, *24*(2), 162-168.

www.ingramcontent.com/pod-product-compliance
Lightning Source LLC
LaVergne TN
LVHW090411210926
848480LV00002B/531
9798348399597